Professional Development

A GUIDE FOR PRIMARY CARE

2nd Edition

Professional Development

A GUIDE FOR PRIMARY CARE

2nd Edition

EDITED BY

Margareth Attwood MSc, DMS, MCIPD
Medical Education Project Manager and Head of National Office
for Summative Assessment, University of Winchester

Anthony Curtis MSc (Dist) Cert Ed
Head of Education and Training, Kennet
and North Wilts PCT and Honorary Lecturer, De Montford University

Dr John Pitts PhD, MSc (Med Ed), MRCGP, FRCGP
Associate Director in Postgraduate GP Education, Wessex Deanery
and Honorary Research Fellow, University of Winchester, and Editor
of *Education for Primary Care*

Dr Robin While MBBS, FRCGP
Severn & Wessex Deanery Lead Associate Director for Avon
Gloucester and Wiltshire Strategic Health Authority/Workforce
Development Confederation

Blackwell
Publishing

First published 2000
Reprinted 2000, 2001
Second edition 2005

Library of Congress Cataloging-in-Publication Data

Data available

ISBN-13: 978-1-4051-2232-0
ISBN-10: 1-4051-2232-3

A catalogue record for this title is available from the British Library

Set in 10/12.75, Minion by TechBooks Inc.
Printed and bound in India by Replika Press Pvt. Ltd.

Commissioning Editor: Alison Brown
Development Editor: Mirjana Misina
Production Controller: Kate Charman

For further information on Blackwell Publishing, visit our website:
http://www.blackwellpublishing.com

The publisher's policy is to use permanent paper from mills that operate a sustainable forestry policy,
and which has been manufactured from pulp processed using acid-free and elementary chlorine-free
practices. Furthermore, the publisher ensures that the text paper and cover board used have met
acceptable environmental accreditation standards.

Contents

List of contributors.. vii

Foreword.. viii

Preface.. ix

List of abbreviations xi

PART 1: GETTING STARTED 1

How to use this workbook 3

The national perspective 4

Background to the NHS 8

Useful websites for *How to use this workbook*.... 10

The practice 12

The practice and links to other organisations ... 12

Review of your current situation 14

National initiatives that have an impact on the

practice 15

nGMS 15

Quality and Outcome Framework (QOF) 16

Clinical Governance.. 17

National Institute of Clinical Excellence............ 20

National Service Frameworks 20

Funding.. 22

Maximising income... 22

Useful websites for *The practice*....................... 25

The patient.. 26

What patients want 26

The Patient Advice and Liaison Service (PALS)

and your practice 27

Gaining patient feedback 28

Using complaints to improve practice.............. 30

New NHS complaint procedure (2004) 31

Useful websites for *The patient*........................ 34

The primary health care team 37

The GP's perspective – counting the 'beans' 37

The practice nurses' perspective 40

Useful websites for *The primary

health care team* 43

PART 2: WHERE DO WE START 45

The practice professional development plan 47

The practice professional development

plan (PPDP).. 47

The personal development plan (PDP)............. 47

What are the best ways to learn?..................... 48

The use of portfolios in learning....................... 48

Reflective practice 49

Local delivery plans and health

needs assessment 52

1 Creating a profile of your

practice population 54

2 Key features of your practice

population... 56

3 Identification of top health problems in

your practice 58

4 Prioritising the list.................................... 62

5 Planning interventions 64

6 Creating an action plan 68

7 New priorities.. 71

Developing the primary health care team.............. 73

Primary health care teams (PHCTs) 73

How to get the most from the PHCT? 73

What are away days?.. 74

Why have away days?....................................... 74

What can be achieved? 74

Away day programme 75

Ground rules for away days 76

Running small groups 76

Tips on running small groups............................ 77

Brainstorming... 77

Practice SCOT analysis..................................... 79

Developing learning profiles for

PHCTs 80

The Learning Styles Helper's Guide 80

Activists 80

Reflectors... 81

Theorists 81

Pragmatists... 81

Reflecting on learning

style questionnaire 82

Skill mix of the primary health care team.............. 83

What is skill mix?... 83

Individual skills assessment (clinical) 84

Individual skills assessment (non-clinical

team members) 86

Team skills assessment 88

Useful websites for *Skill mix of the primary

health care team*.. 92

Appraisal **93**
   GP NHS appraisal 93
   PHCTs appraisal 97
      The heinz medical practice: formal record
      of staff appraisal 100
   360 degrees feedback 103
   Useful websites for *Appraisal* 106

Audit and research **107**
   Research and development (R & D) in primary
   care 107
   Using evidence in the management of common
   diseases 108
      Using evidence in the management of
      common diseases 111
   Practice audit 113
   Significant-event auditing (SEA) 114
      Recording a significant event 117
      Personal sea 118
      Heinz medical practice – recording a
      significant event 119
      Minutes of significant event audit
      meeting – heinz medical practice 121
   Referral data 122
   Prescribing analysis and cost
   (PACT) prescribing 124
      The practice prescribing costs for the last
      quarter 126
   Performance indicators – thinking beyond the
   numbers 128
   Useful websites for *Audit and research* 130

The practice professional
development plan (PPDP) **131**
   Components of the plan 131
      Practice professional development
      plan – the heinz medical practice 132

PART 3: PERSONAL DEVELOPMENT PLAN **135**
Framework for personal
development plans (PDP) **137**
   Getting started 137
      Past educational profile 138
      Learning highlights 140
   The self-audit and personal SCOT analysis 142

Methods of identifying educational needs **144**
   Sticky moments 144
      Discovery page – sticky moments 146
      Identification of educational needs 148

Blind spots 150
Phased evaluation plan (PEP) 150
Phased Evaluation Programme – Question
Bank (PEP-QB) 151
Communication skills 151
Medical ethics 153
Resuscitation 154
Conflict in the consultation – data
entry vs caring 155
Stress and you 158
   Daily stress log at work 160
   Delegation skills checklist 162
Looking after yourself 162
   Managing performance distractors
   self-evaluation 164
   The work of general practice –
   questionnaire 166
Useful websites for *Methods of identifying*
educational needs 173

Meeting educational and
developmental needs **174**
   Learning style 174
   Learning skills – getting the most out of your
   learning 174
   Reflection 175
   Your learning need 175
   Your learning goal 176
   What is available to you 176
   Conclusion 176
   Mentoring 177
   Self-directed learning groups 178
   Keeping up to date 178
   Higher professional education (HPE) 179
   Career pathways 180
   GPs with special interest (GPSIs) 182
   Teaching PCOs 182
   GP retainer and flexible career schemes 183
   GP trainer 185
   For the more adventurous . . .
   career breaks 185
   Useful websites for *Meeting educational*
   and developmental needs 186

Personal development plan **187**
Appendix 1: Confidentiality declaration **191**
Appendix 2: Websites **192**
References and further reading **199**
Index **201**

List of contributors

Ms Sue Bacon
Clinical Governance Support Manager, Kennet and North Wilts PCT

Dr Peter Baskett
Consultant Anaesthetist, Frenchay Hospital, Bristol, Editor of Resuscitation

Mr Arthur Belbin
Director Strategic Planning, West Wiltshire PCT

Mr Brian Canfer
Practice Manager/GP trainer, West Midlands/East Wales

Professor Ruth Chambers
Professor of Primary Care, Centre of Health Policy and Practice, Staffordshire University

Dr Paul Colbrook
Medico Legal Adviser, Medical Defence Union

Professor Colin Coles
Medical Educationalist, University of Winchester

Dr John Elliman
GP and GP Trainer, Swindon

Ms Pam Gates
Freelance Primary Care Trainer and Facilitator; Lay Member of Wessex Deanery, Bath

Ms Ros Grant
Head of Medicines Management, Banes PCT

Dr Michael Greco
Hon Senior Research Fellow in Health Services Research, North Devon RDSU

Dr Phil Hammond
GP returner, writer and broadcaster, Bristol

Dr Anne Hastie
Deputy Dean of Postgraduate GP Education, London Deanery

Ms Naomi Jefferies
Chartered Occupational Psychologist, Bath

Dr Di Jelly
GP, North Shields

Dr David Jenner
GP and NHS Alliance nGMS contract lead, Exeter

Ms Julie Lennon
Education and Training Manager, Kennet and North Wilts PCT

Dr Colin Lennon
GP, Melksham

Dr Murray Lough
Assistant Director (Audit), West of Scotland Deanery

Dr Nick Lyons
Associate Director Postgraduate General Practice Education, Severn and Wessex Deanery

Dr Liz Mearns
Research GP and Clinical Governance Lead, Swindon PCT

Ms Sue Nutbrown
Chair, RCN Practice Nurses Association

Ms Joyce Robins
Director, Patient Concern

Dr Steve Rowlands
Research GP and Associate GP Tutor, Trowbridge

Dr Peter Tate
GP, Corfe Castle

Dr Richard Wharton
GP and GP Tutor, Bath

Dr Vicky Woods
Senior Lecturer, Pan Bath and Swindon Research and Development Unit, University of Bath

Dr John Howard
Associate Director of Postgraduate General Practice Education, Mersey Deanery

Foreword

The Royal College of General Practitioners (RCGP) has led the way in driving up standards in general practice over the last 50 years by setting standards and promoting the education and training of general practitioners (GPs). We are now in a new world where the 'name of the game' for health care professionals is accountability for professional practice and standards to patients, peers, the National Health Service (NHS) and regulators. The landscape has changed totally with the introduction of NHS systems of quality such as clinical governance and appraisals. Nationally we have a system of standard setting through the National Institute for Health and Clinical Excellence (NICE), the national service frameworks and the new GP contract, with its emphasis on an evidence-based quality and outcomes framework.

Getting all this right – and the stakes are high – requires primary health care professionals to have an understanding of policy and techniques for professional development. I know as a practicing GP just how hard it can be to keep up to date in a generalist discipline and showing progress. Just how do you achieve good glycaemic control in a patient with type 2 diabetes faced with a bewildering choice of drugs in the context of the patient's ideas, concerns and expectations? However, it can be done if GP learning of primary care teams is supported properly.

GPs are now in charge of their own learning – since the demise of the postgraduate education allowance in 2003. For many this is a frightening thought: How to plan systematic learning and improvement in the context of a personal and practice professional development plan? It is clear that help is needed for most GPs including 'high achievers' with a process that provides a degree of challenge and stimulation.

GPs want to raise the quality bar even further. As a GP appraiser, I know that the importance and impact of a high-quality learning experience cannot be underestimated. These are however far and few in between! A degree of challenge and sometimes prescription is needed to ensure that GPs remain up to date and fit to practice.

I am convinced that professional development is a process whose potential has not been fully realised and as Chairman of the RCGP, I want to modernise the process. I have no doubt that this book will be a valuable contribution to that modernisation process. We need to take professional development up a notch and to another level – from a superficial process to something deeper and embedded in professional cultures and NHS quality systems.

And so I welcome this book – it is one of the best texts I have read on professional development. I particularly like the emphasis on using tools, audits and forms to inform the professional development planning process. This is a thoughtful book, well researched, up to date and most importantly set in the context of professional development for primary health care professionals in the new and modern NHS.

Preface

Once again the National Health Service (NHS) is changing and along with it comes changes in professional development and the introduction of NHS appraisal and revalidation for general practitioners (GPs). These changes may often bring increased demands but offer new opportunities for personal and professional development, ultimately improving patient care.

Many may find the prospect of revalidation, the process by which GPs will evidence their fitness to practice, as threatening. The way in which revalidation will occur has been debated for several years and the way ahead is still unclear in the months following Dame Janet Smith's Shipman Enquiry. It seems likely, however, that revalidation and GP appraisal will continue with similar evidence being used to inform both processes. This workbook will act as a resource to help individuals in their preparation for these changes.

This workbook will help to provide an educational framework which enables you to plan and structure your continuing professional development and improve quality in general practice. It also provides a framework to meet the requirements of the primary care organisation and clinical governance. It is not an exhaustive list of what can and cannot be achieved, but rather a framework into which you can dovetail your own ideas. In addition, useful website addresses at the end of chapters indicate where further information can be obtained.

We must thank all those who have helped to compile this workbook. We are grateful particularly to those who contributed chapters and responded to the draft version and did the proofreading.

The Editors are grateful to the following for the contribution they made to the First edition of this workbook, which has formed much of the foundation to this volume – Dr Peter Agar; Dr Tim Ballard; Dr Charles Campion-Smith; Mrs Mary Connor; Dr Chris Goldie; Prof Janet Grant; Mrs Kate Harris; Prof Jacky Hayden; Prof Roger Higgs; Dr Claire Kendrick; Dr Roger Kneebone; Mrs Lesley Millard; Prof Mike Pringle; Dr Neil Scheurmier; Dr Paul Smith; Prof Tim Van Zwanenberg; Ms Sarah Walker.

We particularly appreciate the administrative help received from Seana Lamb-Hughes and Rupert Attwood in the compilation of this workbook.

We have been very fortunate in editing this book and to have been offered much advice from Ms Claire Bonnett from Blackwell Publishing. Thanks are also due to Ms Seema Koul, at Techbooks for her invaluable support.

Finally, we are grateful to Kennet and North Wilts PCT, University of Winchester and Astra Zeneca for supporting this production, which we hope will be a valuable and practical guide for all those working in primary care.

Margareth Attwood MSc, DMS, MCIPD
Medical Education Project Manager and Head of National Office
for Summative Assessment, University of Winchester

Anthony Curtis MSc (Dist) Cert Ed
Head of Education and Training, Kennet
and North Wilts PCT and Honorary Lecturer, De Montford University

Dr John Pitts PhD, MSc (Med Ed), MRCGP, FRCGP
Associate Director in Postgraduate GP Education, Wessex Deanery
and Honorary Research Fellow, University of Winchester, and Editor
of *Education for Primary Care*

Dr Robin While MBBS, FRCGP
Severn & Wessex Deanery Lead Associate Director for Avon
Gloucester and Wiltshire Strategic Health Authority/Workforce
Development Confederation

List of abbreviations

BJGP	British Journal of General Practice
BMJ	British Medical Journal
CASP	Critical Appraisal Skills Programme
CFEP	Client Focused Evaluations Programme
CHAI	Commission of Healthcare Audit and Inspection (previous name for Healthcare commission)
CHD	Coronary Heart Disease
CHI	Commission for Health Improvement
CMO	Chief Medical Officer
CNO	Chief Nursing Officer
COAD	Chronic Obstructive Airways Disease
COPD	Chronic Obstructive Pulmonary Disease
COSHH	Control of Substance Hazardous to Health Regulations 2002
CPD	Continuing Professional Development
CPR	Cardio Pulmonary Resuscitation
DISQ	Doctors' Interpersonal Skills Questionnaire
DoH	Department of Health
EBM	Evidence Based Medicine
ECG	Electrocardiogram
ENRiP	Exploring New Roles in Practice
EQUIP	Electronic Quality Information for Patients
GMC	General Medical Council
GMS	General Medical Services
GP	General Practitioner
GPAQ	General Practice Assessment Questionnaire
GPMS	General Practice Medical Services
GPSIs	General Practitioner with a Special interest
GS	Global Sum
HNA	Health Needs Assessment
HPE	Higher Professional Education
HSAW	Health and Safety at Work Regulations 1999
ICAS	Independent Complaints Advocacy Services
ILA	Individual Learning Accounts
IPQ	Improving Practice Questionnaire
IT	Information Technology
JCPTGP	Joint Committee on Postgraduate Training for General Practice
LDPs	Local Delivery Plans
MDU	Medical Defence Union
MI	Myocardial Infarction
MPIG	Minimum Practice Income Guarantee
MRCGP	Member of the Royal College of General Practitioners
nGMS	New GP Contract
NHS	National Health Service
NHSMA	National Health Service Modernisation Agency

NICE	National Institute of Clinical Excellence
NMC	Nursing and Midwifery Council
NPEF	Nurse Prescribers' Extended Formulary
NSF	National Service Framework
PACT	Prescribing Analysis and Cost
PALS	Patient Advice and Liaison Services
PCO	Primary Care Organisation (formerly Groups, Trusts)
PDP	Personal Development Plan
PEP	Phased Evaluation Plan
PGEA	Postgraduate Education Allowance (now defunct!)
PHCT	Primary Health care Team
PI	Performance Indicator
PMS	Personal Medical Services
PPA	Prescription Pricing Authority
PPDP	Practice Professional Development Plan
PPIFs	Patient and Public Involvement Forums
PRIMIS	Primary Care Information Services
QMAS	Quality Management and Analysis System
QOF	Quality and Outcome Framework
R&D	Research and Development
RCGP	Royal College of General Practitioners
RCN	Royal College of Nurses
ScHARR	School of Health and Related Research–University of Sheffield
SCOPME	Standing Committee on Postgraduate Medical and Dental Education
SEA	Significant-Event Auditing
SHAs	Strategic Health Authorities
TRISET	Clinical Terminology browser

PART 1
Getting started

How to use this workbook

This revised and fully updated workbook reflects the work of the whole practice team, building on recent developments for multi-professional working. The new edition of this workbook aims not only to explain what a practice professional development plan (PPDP) and personal development plan (PDP) actually mean, but also to provide a practical approach to bring them to life. GPs and practice staff work 'at the coalface' in the delivery of care to a patient population with ever-increasing demands and expectations. Now, with the added demands of clinical governance, annual appraisal, 5-yearly revalidation and the new GP contract (nGMS), it is hardly surprising that many of us feel overwhelmed.

This workbook may provide the key to meeting the requirements of a PPDP, PDP, clinical governance, appraisal and revalidation all in one go. It takes a 'painting by numbers' approach, starting with local delivery plans, health needs assessment through to the formulation of a PPDP and then, by identifying individual learning needs, to a PDP. It is a menu of opportunities, some of which may seem to be more relevant or useful than others. Significantly, this second edition takes a 'whole systems' approach to working in primary care, updating and reviewing the first edition whilst also building on the strength of the original workbook. It is therefore of direct relevance to all primary health care team (PHCT) staff in different and complementary ways – whether you are a GP, practice nurse, practice manager or support staff.

Each section gives some basic information together with an appropriately completed sample form and a blank form for completion. The nGMS has heralded the demise of the largely discredited Postgraduate Education Allowance (PGEA) scheme, which, although relatively easy to administer, was based on the number of hours spent attending educational activity, rather than identifying the individuals' educational needs and drawing up an educational plan.

Research shows that this approach is much more likely to change clinical practice and improve health care. It is consistent with the requirement of the nGMS in which GPs are rightly focused on participating in their annual primary care organisations (PCOs) appraisal and meeting the criteria for revalidation. This workbook provides all the reference material necessary to complete GP PCO appraisal documentation as well as to conduct practice staff appraisals.

It proposes that the PPDP is the starting point, although a PDP is just as important. It is recommended that an individual PDP should relate in some way to the PPDP. If, for example, a practice identifies a need to provide an in-house rheumatology service and no one in the PHCT has the skills and knowledge to take the lead, someone in the team would need to include it in their PDP. This could, for example, state that they were planning to study for an MSc in primary care rheumatology by distance learning. Each member of the PHCT could offer to become a resource for the practice by taking on something from the PPDP into his/her PDP. Sessional doctors (locum, salaried doctor, retainer, flexible career scheme doctor and GP registrar) and other staff (e.g. nurse practitioners, practice nurses, health visitors, community nurses, managers, audit clerks, healthcare assistants, receptionists, dispensers) working regularly in the practice should also be included. All team members will of course have different, though complementary, learning needs and plans for the future. This workbook attempts to show how these needs might be identified and discusses various methods of meeting these needs. There is also a reminder about the importance of certain generic skills, knowledge and attitudes – such as consultation skills, resuscitation, medical ethics and 'looking after yourself', which are so important for everyone who works in PHCTs.

To quote from the *Gestalt Law of Pragnanz*, 'The whole is more than the sum of its parts'. This is surely true in primary care where the practice (the whole) is more than the sum of the individual GPs and members of the PHCT that comprise it. This should be borne in mind when formulating both a PPDP and a PDP. It is very important to reflect on the relationships between the parts, not just the parts themselves, in considering overall practice and practice staff effectiveness.

The national perspective

This framework for professional development was inspired by the Chief Medical Officer's report *A Review of Continuing Professional Development in General Practice 1998*, emphasising a high premium on quality in the National Health Service (CMO 1998). The pursuit of quality can be broken down into three distinct but interrelated strands:
- clinical governance;
- enhanced professional self-regulation; and
- lifelong learning.

Clinical governance is a system through which NHS organisations are accountable for continuously improving the quality of their services and safeguarding high standards of care by creating an environment in which excellence in clinical care will flourish. Continuing professional development (CPD) is one of the central components of clinical governance and can be defined as:

> A process of lifelong learning for all individuals and teams which enables professionals to expand and fulfil their potential and which also meets the needs of patients and delivers the health and health care priorities of the NHS.

The traditional model of PGEA had fundamental weaknesses. Often the learning methods were inappropriate and the evaluation of its impact was, in general, rudimentary. There was fragmentation among different groups within primary care, leading to difficulty in achieving a coordinated approach to education. The vision of the CMO's report identified three interested parties:
- the profession;
- the patients;
- the NHS.

CPD needs to be seen in this context. The concept of CPD is relatively new in the field of medicine but has been used extensively and successfully elsewhere.

What is professional development?

Right from the outset, it is important to understand what we mean by 'professional development'. Rather surprisingly, many of the interventions in recent years have not been fully thought through, nor have been entirely explicit about the nature of professional practice and how it develops. They have not always presented the (again surprisingly large) literature that forms the evidence base for professional development. This section looks at some of the concepts involved and presents some of the evidence.

To try to understand professional development we will briefly try to answer four key questions:

- What is professional practice?
- What is professional knowledge?
- How does practice change naturally?
- How can natural change be fostered?

What is professional practice?

Anyone entering a profession adopts what Golby and Parrott (1999) call 'a tradition of conduct'. As Carr (1995) puts it:

> To 'practise' . . . is always to act within a tradition, and it is only by submitting to its authority that practitioners can begin to acquire the practical knowledge and standards of excellence by means of which their own practical competence can be judged. (pp. 68–9)

Carr claims that this form of practice:

> . . . can only be made intelligible in terms of the inherited and largely unarticulated body of practical knowledge which constitutes the tradition within which the good intrinsic to a practice is enshrined. (p. 68)

Epstein (1999) notes that much professional practice is 'unconscious'. Experienced clinicians, he says:

> . . . apply to their practice a large body of knowledge, skill, values, and experiences that are not explicitly stated by or known to them . . . While explicit elements of practice are taught formally, tacit elements are usually learned during observation and practice. Often excellent clinicians are less able to articulate what they do than others who observe them . . . Evidence-based medicine (EBM) offers a structure for analysing medical decision-making, but it is not sufficient to describe the more tacit process of expert clinical judgement. (p. 834)

Professional practice means dealing with difficult, complex problems that are often 'indeterminate' (Schön 1984). It is concerned with 'the swampy lowlands' (Schön 1984), and requires 'reading the situation' (Fish & Coles 1998), being flexible, and (perhaps surprisingly for those who believe exclusively in EBM) *improvising*.

Gawande (2002), in his very useful book *Complications: A Surgeon's Notes on an Imperfect Science*, says that 'these are the moment in which medicine actually happens' (p. 7). He adds:

> We look for medicine to be an orderly field of knowledge and procedure. But it is not. It is an imperfect science, an enterprise of constantly changing knowledge, uncertain information, fallible individuals, and at the same time lives on the line. There is science

in what we do . . . but also habit, intuition and sometimes plain old guessing. The gap between what we know and what we aim for persists. And this gap complicates everything we do . . . [Medicine is] what happens when the simplicities of science come up against the complexities of individual lives. (pp. 7–8)

This certainly has an implication for the development of protocols, which are devised to determine what professionals should do in *routine* cases. What Schön is saying (and many others agree) is that the expertise of the professional comes into being *in situations where protocols can no longer apply* (which, as doctors recognise, is most of the time!).

But becoming a *caring* professional also means accepting a commitment to some form of human welfare:

The kind of work [caring professionals do] is . . . especially important for the well-being of individuals or of society at large, having a value so special that money cannot serve as its sole measure; it is . . . 'Good Work'. (Freidson 1994, p. 200)

What is professional knowledge?

The General Medical Council (1993) recognises much of this when it notes that one of the attributes of the independent medical practitioner is:

The capacity to solve clinical and other problems in medical practice, which involves or requires: (i) an intellectual and temperamental ability to change, to face the unfamiliar and to adapt to change; (ii) a capacity for individual, self-directed learning; and (iii) reasoning and judgement in the application of knowledge to the analysis and interpretation of data, in defining the nature of a problem, and in planning and implementing a strategy to resolve it. (p. 25)

Professional practice in health care, then, is a *moral endeavour* – it fundamentally involves the capacity of someone to engage in 'right' action in human situations, where there is often no 'absolute' or 'correct' answer, but only that which engages the professional in 'that form of wise and prudent judgement which takes account of what would be morally appropriate in a particular situation'. Professional action can only be considered 'right' then, in the sense that it is based on 'reasoned action that can be defended discursively in argument and justified as morally appropriate to the particular circumstances in which it was taken' (Carr 1995, pp. 70–71).

Eraut (1994) distinguishes between different kinds of professional knowledge, noting that factual (or as he calls it 'propositional') knowledge is only part of what informs professional action. Professionals also possess 'personal knowledge', which is acquired through experience. As we have already seen, other writers agree (Epstein 1999; Gawande 2002).

Carr (1995) distinguishes between human actions that on the one hand lead to making something (which requires a form of knowledge the Greeks called *techne*, which today we would call 'technical knowledge'), and on the other hand lead to people's moral judgements (which requires a special kind of knowledge – *phronesis*, which today we would translate as 'practical wisdom').

Professional knowledge, then, is:

. . . not a way of resolving technical problems for which there is, in principle, some correct answer. Rather it is a way of resolving those moral dilemmas which occur when different ethically desirable ends entail different, and perhaps incompatible, courses of action. (pp. 70–71)

How does professional practice change naturally?

Much of the practical wisdom needed for professional practice is acquired 'naturally', that is by professional people 'absorbing and being absorbed into a community of practice' (Lave & Wenger 1991). This occurs largely through the everyday conversations professionals have with one another, through them learning *from* talk as well as learning *to* talk. In short, professionals are 'socialised' into the traditions of their practice.

To say, however, that professionals enter into a tradition does not imply that professional practice is merely 'passed on' uncritically from one generation to the next. It is not 'mechanically or passively reproduced' (Carr 1995, p. 69). As Carr notes, 'the authoritative nature of a tradition doesn't make it immune to criticism' (p. 69). Rather, he argues, a key principle of 'being professional' is that professionals ensure that their practice is 'constantly being reinterpreted and revised through dialogue and discussion about how to pursue the practical goods which constitute the tradition' (p. 69). Epstein (1999) calls this 'mindful practice'.

Carr's argument is that this 'capacity' for changing one's practice is developed through what he calls 'critical reconstruction'. This is a process through which 'a tradition evolves and changes rather than remains static and fixed' (p. 69). He warns that someone who lacks this capacity for critical reconstruction 'may be technically accountable, but . . . can never be morally answerable' (p. 71). He also sees this as a corporate process where 'the collective deliberation of the many is always preferable to the isolated deliberation of the individual' (p. 71).

This implies that the caring professional is not just someone with technical expertise, nor someone capable of making prudent judgements in complex, indeterminate situations (Eraut 1994; Schön 1984) where there is a moral concern for others. It also suggests that professionals engage in the 'critical reconstruction' of their practice, that is they 'deliberate' on their practice so as to defend and justify their judgements in light of the particular circumstances in which they were made.

This, therefore, clarifies the aims of professional education – it is not simply a technical updating of competence (although technical competence is important too), but a constant renewal of one's capacity to make professional judgements. Furthermore, it clarifies the fact that professional people, *because they are professionals*, seek constantly to refine their practice. Throughout their careers, doctors are learning and refining this capacity to change *through their practice*.

How can natural change be fostered?

So, change is natural for professionals, but it does not always happen. Why is this? A Standing Committee on Postgraduate Medical and Dental Education (SCOPME) report (1998a) on CPD suggested a number of reasons:

- pressures of service work;
- inappropriate work tasks;
- education not being valued or rewarded;
- no feedback or review (SCOPME 1999); and
- the colleges' points systems.

Clearly, any new CPD interventions must not merely re-invent the same wonky wheel! But what *should* happen? SCOPME suggests the following:

- people's needs must be voiced;
- a balance of personal, professional and working life;
- development should be recognised and valued;
- there should be local analysis of problems and solutions;
- mentor's skills need developing (SCOPME 1998b);
- CPD schemes should be evaluated;
- CPD should not be related to monitoring, accreditation, remuneration or promotion; and
- organisational support should be given.

Further insight comes from the Government's White Paper on quality *A First Class Service* (NHS 1998a). In its definition of 'clinical governance' there is the following suggestion as to how quality can be established:

> . . . by creating an environment in which excellence in health care will flourish. (NHS 1998a, p. 33)

There is in this phrase a biological, even botanical, imagery. We all know about environments that lead to things flourishing: nurture, nutrients, warmth and support. (We also know about environments where things do not flourish: hostile, overcrowded, lacking in basic life support).

Natural development is more likely to occur in a supportive environment, and CPD arrangements should facilitate this. This workbook seeks to meet this objective.

Background to the NHS

Some readers may find this summary describing the background and structures of the NHS useful.

The NHS was founded in 1948 and is now the largest employer in Europe and one of the largest employers in the world next to the Chinese Army and the Indian Railways. It comprises more than 1.3 million staff working in more than 40 different occupational groups (the NHS is clearly more than just doctors and nurses).

The NHS is financed mainly through taxation and, therefore, relies on Parliament for its funding. It is accountable through the Secretary of State for Health – the Cabinet member responsible for the service. As a result, the government has to publicly explain and defend its policies for the NHS.

The Department of Health (DoH) has overall responsibility for the NHS and its purpose is to support the government to improve the health and well-being of the population. In order to do this they have devised the NHS Plan, a radical 10-year action plan (1995–2005) setting out a wide range of measures to put patients and people at the heart of our health and social services.

The National Health Service Modernisation Agency (NHSMA) was established in April 2001 to support the NHS and its partner organisations in modernising services to meet the needs and convenience of patients. Its focus has been mainly on improving access, increasing local support, raising standards and dissemination of knowledge. The NHSMA works closely with Strategic Health Authorities (SHAs) that, amongst other responsibilities, performance-manage PCOs so that they can implement and deliver the NHS Plan. SHAs are also responsible for creating a coherent strategic NHS framework, building capacity and supporting performance improvement.

There are 28 SHAs (each covering an average population of 1.8 million people) responsible for developing strategies for local health services and ensuring high-quality performance (see the following flow chart on the Structure of the NHS). They manage the NHS locally and are a key link between the DoH and the NHS front line. They also ensure that national priorities (such as programmes for improving cancer services) are integrated into Local Delivery Plans.

STRUCTURE OF THE NHS

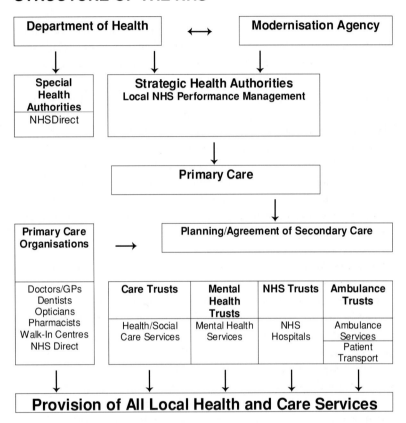

A total of 303 PCOs (each serving an average population of 170,000 people) are the cornerstone of the NHS locally (comprising 75% of the total NHS budget). They run primary and community care services and also commission secondary care. Their main functions are to improve the health of the community (e.g. assessing health needs, tackling health inequalities and leading partnership working with local authorities). PCOs are also responsible for commissioning all acute and specialised care, as well as services for mental health, emergency ambulances and patient transport, NHS-Direct and walk-in centres. They also implement population-screening programmes. PCOs work collaboratively, involving patients and the public as well as their own GP practices and partners. They coordinate agencies charged with the responsibility of the delivery of health care, creating strong local partnerships and working across traditional boundaries in the delivery of health and social care.

PCOs also make most of the commissioning (i.e. purchasing) decisions based on a health needs assessment of their local service as well as patient numbers and user population. They then work with potential health care providers to develop a service to meet those needs. Commissioned services could range from a state-of-the-art new hospital scanner to provision of meals-on-wheels service for the elderly. Joint commissioning of services by PCOs (i.e. health care) and social services (i.e. social care) allows a more strategic and 'joined-up' approach to the planning and delivery of services to the same users, whilst also using resources collaboratively in order to achieve the best outcomes. However, PCOs and social services are at different stages of integration across the UK and only a minority have developed into 'full-integration' (i.e. care trusts) – one statutory organisation delivering both services.

Primary care is where approximately 90% of NHS patients receive their treatment, resulting in more than 250 million appointments being made every year. The NHS Plan promised that by December 2004 all patients would be seen by a GP within two working days or by a primary care professional within one working day. As the flow chart shows, primary care involves the interface of GP practices with PCOs, care trusts, mental health-care trusts, NHS trusts and ambulance trusts, all of which are involved in complementary yet different ways in improving local health care and social care services. Advances in health care, especially in diagnostics and minor surgery, mean that many more treatments that used to be carried out in hospitals can now be performed in primary care. This is more convenient to patients in particular and the NHS in general. The GP surgery is of course the focus of most primary care, and the range of services offered here continues to expand.

In addition, there are now 43 walk-in centres throughout England that provide fast access to advice and treatment for minor ailments and injuries without appointments. These walk-in centres are open 7 days a week, from early morning to late evening, and offer assessment by experienced NHS nurses as well as provide information on out-of-hours, GP, dental and local pharmacy services.

Some large primary care centres now include GPs, dentists, opticians, health visitors, pharmacists and social workers, all working together often in multi-agency teams in order to deliver the best quality and range of services to patients. In addition, a national telephone helpline service, NHSDirect, is staffed by health care professionals and can be contacted on

0845 46 47

Useful websites for *How to use this workbook*

Department of Health (DoH)	www.doh.gov.uk
NHSDirect	www.nhsdirect.nhs.uk
NHS in England – Gateway to NHS Organisations	http://www.nhs.uk/england/ default.aspx
National Health Service Modernisation Agency	www.modern.nhs.uk www.dh.gov.uk
NHS Walk-In Centres	www.nhs.uk/England/ noAppointmentNeeded/ walkinCentres/default.aspx

A full list of websites can be found on pages 192–197.

QUESTIONS

Given the previous article, what changes would you like to see in the way that your practice delivers services so that they maximise choice, value and quality to your patients?

How may you and/or your PHCT maximise your/their own understanding of the NHS structure and functions as a result of this initiative?

What learning and/or development opportunities for staff are there in your practice?

The practice

The practice and links to other organisations

Very few people working in health care can now work alone. Much greater achievements can be made by teams than individuals and it is recognised that we also will be far more successful if we work with other organisations to create the best outcome for our patients. Some of this working may be formalised, e.g. provision of a service through an agreed service level agreement, whilst other work may be less formal, e.g. the practice supporting a local weight-loss initiative.

Links with primary care organisations (PCOs)

Whilst the PHCT prepare their own practice professional development plans (PPDPs) and personal development plans (PDPs) and review their function, your practice is part of a larger organisation – PCO. The aspiration of good health, and access to care for all, can only occur if all levels of the PCO work effectively in partnership together. This is not always easy. The steer from above is likely to be driven by funding (we all want to be paid). The reflections from below are not always as easy to flag up, but the process of reviewing quality through clinical governance and the aspirations in a PPDP both present opportunities to do so. The process of practice-based commissioning will also create a situation where local priorities can be addressed.

Priorities, of course, mean choices. This means that some things cannot be achieved. Decision-making needs information and evidence, some of which will be found in conjunction with your PCO. There are a number of ways in which practices will link with PCOs regarding quality of care. Many of these are informal but increasingly they have a statutory basis.

- New GP contract (nGMS) or personal medical services (PMS) contract.
- Clinical governance.
- Medicines management.
- Practice-based commissioning.
- Education provision.

> When considering the practices relationship with the PCO it is probably useful to consider some of the dilemmas faced in the relationship:
> - Performance management vs development
> - Quality vs cost
> - Assessment vs support
>
> Understanding each other's roles is key to a good relationship between practices and PCOs.

Links with education

There are various bodies other than PCOs that provide and advise on education for health professionals. Closely related to many is their professional body, e.g. Royal College of General Practitioners (RCGP) or Royal College of Nurses (RCN) and the local deanery structure, that organises educational networks for GPs in local areas. There are also elements of the National Health Service Modernisation Agency (NHSMA) and workforce development parts of the NHS that provide education to a wider range of professionals that practices can effectively use. Education is also facilitated by some charitable organisations (usually specific to their area of concern) and by drug companies. Secondary care trusts and the specialists working in them will also provide a source of educational help.

Each of these groups can help practices find answers to specific needs in different ways. The form of learning will vary but very often the process is very much a two-way affair, with all parties contributing to discussions not so much about how to do things right but about how collectively to do them better.

> It is an important part of personal and practice development to work out how you can best contribute to the process. As well as linking with the various organisations to learn from their expertise, you need to link with them so that they can also learn from yours.

Links with other NHS organisations

Increasingly the NHS is becoming a unified system of provision. The practice will receive prescribing analysis and cost (PACT) information from the Prescription Pricing Authority and will be expected to be conversant with the guidance of the National Institute of Clinical Excellence. It will also need to consider the proposals in the National Service Frameworks.

Links with other local and national organisations

As practice-based commissioning develops, there will be more need to have explicit links with district hospitals as well as the long-standing informal links with specialists. Practices cannot function in isolation. Much closer links with social services mean that connections with those teams are closer and bringing benefits. You will also know about other local organisations that help the same patients, clients and users as you.

There are national organisations such as the Citizens Advice Bureau and those that help carers and older people, or patients with specific diseases. There are those that provide central facilities for the old or mentally ill, and those that help with local transport arrangements that may be part of national or local organisations.

Many PCOs were arranged to have shared boundaries with those of local authorities and whilst most links with them will occur at that level, there are many community subdivisions with an interest in the health and social care needs of the same population. Some of the concerning issues to practices will be the same as those of community groups especially in areas where major demographic changes in employment or population occur.

Example

A local charitable organisation helped patients by bringing them to the surgery for their appointments. It was finding that it did not have enough drivers to cover all the requests made and so was having to plan to be selective about who it helped. Some patients not helped with transport were then likely to ask for house calls. The situation was discussed with the practice manager of the surgery who suggested that some appointments were allocated to patients brought in by the scheme drivers. By having two such appointments together and alerting the doctors to them it became easy to ensure that they were not kept waiting too long. The drivers could then pick up two people at once and not have to wait at the surgery, allowing them to be able to do another journey the same morning. The benefits to both sides were obvious after only a short time.

REVIEW OF YOUR CURRENT SITUATION

Which organisations are concerned with the same people as you?

With which of those organisations do you share similar aims?

Can you help any other organisations?

How would you do so?

Can any other organisations help you?

How would they do so?

Can you work more closely with some organisations to gain mutual benefit?

If so, how can this be achieved?

National initiatives that have an impact on the practice
The new GP contract (nGMS)

The philosophy behind the nGMS contract was to reward good quality care and at the same time allow the practice some choice in the services offered. A number of services had been devolved to primary care without the financial support for their implementation. This resulted in an overload of work which made general practice unattractive and consequently recruiting and retaining staff became difficult. The government recognises that primary care is where approximately 90% of the total health care is delivered. There was an urgent need to address this dichotomy and the nGMS contract was the result. *Essential* services had never been defined. There was a strong feeling among GPs that core services should be clearly and comprehensively defined; however, this was not achieved in the negotiations. Therefore, the potential remains for a similar situation to develop if practitioners do not objectively assess proposed future developments and decide if they want to undertake the work (and whether they will be able or unable to deliver a cost-effective quality service).

Briefly, the basic elements of the nGMS contract are as follows:

Funding streams
- The global sum (GS) is subject to a minimum practice income guarantee (MPIG) which ensures it is not less than the historic global sum equivalent.
- Payments from the PCO are no longer made quarterly and do not depend upon the submission of claims from the practice. The majority of practice income comes from *essential* and *additional* services and is contained in the GS/MPIG, which is paid monthly in advance. Funding allocations are agreed annually by the PCO at the start of the financial year although this amount may be adjusted during the year according to list size changes, etc. Other funding streams include PCO administered funds, e.g. enhanced services and quality payments, seniority allowance, premises, information management/ technology and dispensing.

Essential services

In essence, these are concerned with the management of registered patients and temporary residents who are:
- Ill but expected to recover.
- Terminally ill.
- Experiencing chronic disease.

The management of these patients are determined by the practice in discussion with the patient.

Additional services

The contract also discusses additional services that practices can agree to provide, payment being included within the GS/MPIG. The practice can opt out or make alternative arrangements for these without formally opting out.

These additional services include:
- Vaccinations and immunisations.
- Childhood immunisations and boosters.
- Curettage, cautery and cryotherapy.

Some additional services also attract payments for achieving targets in the form of points under the Quality and Outcome Framework:

15

- Cervical screening.
- Child health surveillance.
- Maternity services (non-intrapartum).
- Contraceptive services.

Enhanced services

- Directed enhanced services
  - Access.
  - Childhood vaccinations and immunisations.
  - Influenza vaccination.
  - Minor surgery.
  - Quality information preparation.
  - Violent patients.

  All these are funded individually and the practice can decide whether to offer the service or not. In the future it is envisaged that this will lead to some rationalisation and practices that are able to offer a cost-effective quality model may be able to offer services across their local area. Conversely, practices may find that they lose the opportunity to offer a service that they had hitherto provided.
- National enhanced services
  - Anticoagulation monitoring.
  - Intrapartum care.
  - Intrauterine contraceptive device fitting.
  - Minor injury services.
  - More specialised services for patients with multiple sclerosis.
  - More specialised sexual health services.
  - Patients who are alcohol and/or drug misusers.
  - Provision of near-patient testing, e.g. blood testing for methotrexate.
  - Provision of immediate care and first response care.
  - Specialised care of patients with depression.
- Local enhanced services

  There is scope here for negotiation between the provider (practice) and the PCO to offer further services that have been highlighted by local health needs assessment and may include:
  - Cover for a local community hospital.
  - Provision of additional services to an opted out practice.
  - Running adolescence health clinics at local schools.

Quality and Outcome Framework (QOF)

Four domains have been agreed that will attract enhanced payments according to the attainment of stipulated clinical and organisational indicators identified as points. These are:

1   **Patient experience**

    The government has stipulated that the patients' experience of primary care services should be audited by the practice. They have set the length of the routine booked appointment at not less than 10 minutes. The practice should undertake an approved annual survey, reflect on the results and propose changes if appropriate. They should also discuss their results with either a patient group or a non-executive director of the PCO. They will be required to provide some evidence that the changes have been implemented. Patients should expect equal access to quality care because of the universal baseline benchmarking of quality.

2 **Out of Hours Arrangements**

GPs no longer have 24-hour responsibility for their patients. PCOs are now charged with providing medical care for all patients in their area from 1830 hours to 0800 hours Monday to Friday and from 1830 hours Friday until 0800 hours Monday and all bank holidays. Practices must agree as a whole to opt in or to opt out.

3 **Pensions**

This is the government's second main driver, which it is hoped will improve recruitment. All NHS work will now be pensionable, e.g. clinical assistant, locum work, community hospital cover. The **dynamising factor** will also be uplifted. During the contract introduction period, it is generally not advisable for GPs to consider retiring before April 2006 because of the effect of the dynamising factor on likely increasing income streams during this period.

4 **Seniority payments**

The new scheme will offer a 30% increase on current seniority payments, which recognises the working commitment of GPs and uses superannuable income as the measure of that commitment.

Clinical governance

Central to the nGMS is the notion of clinical governance which is the name for established concepts of quality of care. It is about finding ways to make things better, and improve quality for you, your practice, your patients and their carers. Clinical governance is a framework through which NHS organisations are accountable for continuously improving the quality of their services and safeguarding high standards of care by creating an environment in which excellence in clinical care will flourish (NHS Plan 2000).

Clinical governance is a way of continually improving our services so that more patients:

- receive treatments that are based on evidence-based medicine; and
- do not wait so long to receive their treatment.

Moreover, it leads to:

- a reduction in adverse incidents;
- better patient–clinical relationship;
- improved patient care pathways
- improved cooperation and coordination between managers; and
- overall patient satisfaction.

It is important that as professionals and individuals we look to our own individual practice and the contribution this makes to clinical governance and, therefore, the quality of care we provide.

Clinical governance means:

- Establishing robust systems and processes in all areas of your work.
- Seeking opportunities from which we can learn and improve. It is about learning from mistakes and near misses, establishing what went wrong and recognising that it is often a series of events that lead to mistakes. It is therefore crucial to ensure that effective processes or systems are in place to prevent errors happening.
- Working together, developing teams and using everyone's unique talents to work together cooperatively. It incorporates views of patients and enables them to participate in developing and changing services to provide good quality care to support their needs.

- Creating an open and questioning culture
- Monitoring, evidencing and evaluating what you do

GP practices will be required to demonstrate that they meet the Standards for Better Health (Health Care Commission, 2005) which include the following 7-domains:

1 Safety
2 Clinical and Cost Effectiveness
3 Governance
4 Patient Focus
5 Accessible and Responsive Care
6 Care Environment and Amenities
7 Public Health

Within each of these domains, there are both core and developmental standards to achieve. Further information on these can be accessed from 'Assessment for Improvement: The Annual Health Check (2005). London: Health Care Commission.'

What can we do as an individual/team/practice to ensure we embrace the clinical governance umbrella?

1 We can ensure we **support and involve patients** by:
   - inviting them to be involved in planning services;
   - developing relationships with 'expert patients';
   - involving them in groups and obtaining feedback, e.g. with PCO, acute trusts, etc.;
   - offering them a choice in access to services and treatment;
   - identifying the needs and recognise the rights of those who use our services, and address them appropriately; and
   - engaging them in practice work, e.g. involving them in planning audits, in designing information leaflets, in support networks, in 360 degree appraisals and in information sourcing.

2 We can **reduce risk** by:
   - identifying and managing risks and using risk assessments;
   - ensuring we have policies, procedures and systems in place to minimise risks, e.g. dealing with difficult patients, health and safety, control of infection, handwashing, training GP registrars for use of equipment, medicine management, waste disposal, etc.;
   - using near misses, critical incidents, significant events and complaints to learn from and prevent reoccurrence; and
   - feeding back to colleagues, partners and people we work with when things have gone wrong or worked very well.

3 We can **support staff** in their roles by:
   - treating them with respect and dignity regardless of their position;
   - employing staff at the appropriate grades;
   - developing staff through appraisal and training;
   - incorporating them in the practice team;
   - involving staff in business planning and the PPDP;
   - encouraging them to network with their peers; and
   - supporting their personal and professional development.

4 We can ensure **staff will be competent** to the practice by:
   - developing clinical supervision structures (reflective supervision, mentoring, peer review, competency review, etc.);
   - actively engaging in continuing professional development and life-long learning;

- ensuring all staff have annual appraisals, which identify training needs, review job descriptions and have ongoing PDPs;
- supporting staff to enhance their practice through research, audit, networking and learning;
- managing poor performance; and
- ensuring that managerial and clinical leadership responsibilities and accountabilities are clear.

5 We can ensure we are **clinically effective** by:
- being prepared to learn from others;
- using research findings to enhance and develop practice;
- reflecting on our practice;
- developing critical appraisal skills;
- using robust, up-to-date and clinically effective guidelines;
- developing evidence-based practice;
- working in a multidisciplinary way;
- undertaking meaningful and multidisciplinary audit;
- implementing change as a result of regular audits and their findings;
- sharing good practice; and
- ensuring patients receive services promptly.

6 We can ensure that we use our **information systems** effectively and efficiently by:
- collecting robust patient information and having accurate disease registers in place;
- implementing systems to review prescribing and medicines management prescription and management of medicines;
- adhering to Caldicott, the Freedom of Information and Data Protection Acts;
- ensuring staff have access to the Internet and evidence-based websites;
- enabling staff to develop competent IT skills;
- collecting timely information for QOF reviews; and
- using public health information to promote, protect and improve the health of our population.

Both clinical governance and local delivery plans are activities that need grass root input as well as National Service Framework input: 'top down' as well as 'bottom up'. The health needs assessment and clinical audit activities within your practice development will provide this vital 'grass roots' information, whilst the practice-based initiatives are often the product of national 'top down' inputs (e.g. National Service Framework targets), priorities and targets.

Recent local 'bottom up' initiatives have involved GPs working together across traditional practice boundaries in tackling a shared community health problem (substance misuse), using the first edition of this workbook as a vehicle for interpractice collaboration.

Example

Your practice's health needs assessment has identified substance misuse as a local problem. Substance misusers play GPs and practices against one another, and the response is inconsistent. You perceive a need to examine this problem and report this to the clinical governance group via your practice clinical governance lead.

The local GP tutor responds to this educational need and convenes a study workshop to examine the best way of dealing with this in the local area. The workshop reports its conclusions to the PCO, and the clinical governance group gathers information from all local practices about range and scale of problems. The PCO responds with a local management plan and guidelines, and reports this to the partnership board, which then includes a section on substance misuse in the local delivery plan.

With resources targeted to these problems, GPs and their teams are assisted by substance misuse advisers and start to address the problem in a consistent and effective way.

 How can you *demonstrate* that you have provided the best possible care in the best way to your patients?

National Institute of Clinical Excellence (NICE)

Another clinical governance issue concerns equality of access to the best quality care. The perception was that access and provision of health care was based on a 'postcode lottery'. To address this concern, NICE was established in 1999 to make national recommendations of best practices across England and Wales.

It focuses on the whole process of health care delivery and prevention in primary and secondary care. It concentrates on areas where there are confusion and wide discrepancies in approach, or lack of evidence to guide clinical management. It does not investigate all new treatments. Areas for review are selected by the government; however, individuals or organisations can suggest topics to NICE for investigation.

National Service Frameworks (NSFs)

A related national initiative around promoting clinical excellence was the establishment of NSFs, the first of which were launched in 1998. These are evidence-based programmes setting quality standards and specifying services to be available for a particular condition or care group.

Each NSF establishes key requirements:
- National standards and key interventions for a defined group.
- Strategies to support implementation.
- Audit cycles.
- Measures to raise quality and reduce variations in service provision from area to area.

Usually only one new NSF is released in a year. The programme so far covers:

1 Mental Health – 1999
2 Diabetes – Standards – 1999
3 Coronary Heart Disease – 2000
4 National Cancer Plan – 2000
5 Older People – 2001
6 Renal Services – 2004
7 Long-Term Conditions – 2004
8 Children – 2004

The full impact of the NICE recommendations and NSF implementation is yet to be realised. However, the following are areas to be considered when planning to undertake the work:

1 **Patient expectation, positive as well as negative and informed dissent from recommended treatment**

   With greater access to information, many patients are now aware of what treatment and opportunities should be available for them. There are many examples of a disparity between what is desirable and the realities of good clinical practice and budgets.

2 Staffing expertise

The staff who are expected to carry out the recommendations need to have appropriate training to ensure their expertise is evidence based and up to date. There will be a need for investment of time and money by the practice in developing the skills required. It is important to look closely at the skill mix of both clinicians and administrative staff to maximise the potential resource. Increased profitability under the new contract depends very much on minimising unnecessary expenditure.

3 Capacity

It was expected that the work would happen within the current working schedule. The implementation of the nGMS is an attempt to address this imbalance.

The increased monitoring required places an added burden on the practice and it is advisable at the planning stage to adjust the skill mix to achieve a cost-effective service. The role of the health care assistant has broadened in the face of this imperative and it is worth exploring ways of maximising their role, e.g. blood pressures, ECGs, screening, as well as phlebotomy. A national register of the health care assistant has also recently been established to ensure that fitness for practice is maintained.

4 Secondary care limitations

The limitation imposed by the interface with secondary care is largely beyond the PHCTs control, but can make a significant impact on their ability to comply with the recommendations.

Adherence to strict time recommendations within the guidelines is sometimes made difficult when parts of the service are outside the control of the PHCT. An example of this is new cancers. Newly suspected cancer patients should have their first appointment with the specialist within 2 weeks of the referral. Not all hospital trusts are able to deliver this. It is wise for GPs to become involved in the process of developing disease pathways. Steering groups are set up to address specific topics and meet to agree the disease pathway that will facilitate the patients' journey, bridging the interface between primary and secondary care whilst improving the outcome for the patient.

One solution explored is the shift from secondary to primary care of services capable of being delivered just as well, or sometimes more effectively, e.g. community echocardiogram service. This is not a perfect solution as it is bound by some of the same constraints, i.e. skill and resources currently experienced in secondary care. Another approach is adopted in practice-based commissioning and pilots are currently underway.

5 Prescribing

The 'Traffic Light System' clarifies clear parameters of responsibility for primary care clinicians and is a good example of where communication has been developed, which leads to improved health care. 'Green light drugs' can be prescribed and monitored wholly in primary care. 'Amber light drugs' are generally initiated in secondary care and monitored there until the patient is stable. The responsibility can then be transferred to primary care at the request of the consultant. This request should always be accompanied by clear written information about the drug, its side effects and interactions and monitoring requirements before the GP accepts responsibility. Red light drugs should only be initiated in secondary care and it is usual for the prescribing responsibilities to remain the remit of the specialist.

Practices need to effectively manage their prescribing budgets; however, these budgets may well increase when the true disease prevalence is clear.

The 'also-rans'. It is important that everyone is aware that there is the potential for certain patient groups to become disadvantaged. Where the drive to quality is through financial reward it is inevitable that groups not featured in the NSFs may attract less attention than they deserve.

> ? A practice that has spent time and effort in producing an accurate disease register (e.g. hypertension) will be spending far more on cardiovascular drugs than a practice that has yet to identify all their hypertensive patients. Which is the better practice?

Funding
The whole thrust of the nGMS, NICE and NSFs is a quality expectation that the poorer performers will match the standards of the best. By implication this means that there will be a quantity of new work that was not previously being addressed, carrying with it significant funding implications that have not been quantified neither centrally nor locally. This is exemplified by the increased cost of monitoring patients with chronic disease.

It is yet to be realised who the poorer performers are. It is hoped that the new contract will provide the objective evidence that has hitherto been lacking. Until then, subjective judgements are being made purely in terms of quantity: for example, practices are being expected to stay within budgets that are unrealistic and not having been based on any objective knowledge of disease prevalence.

Maximising income
The importance of data quality (particularly with payments for QOF points within the nGMS being linked to data recording on clinical systems) is vital to ensure your practice makes the most of its income.

The nGMS contract provides a major focus on **quality and outcomes** and seeks to reward practices for delivering quality care with extra incentives to encourage even higher standards in four main components focusing on:
- **Clinical standards** covering coronary heart disease, stroke or transient ischaemic attacks, hypertension, diabetes, chronic obstructive pulmonary disease, epilepsy, cancer, mental health, hypothyroidism and asthma.
- **Organisational standards** covering records and information about patients, information for patients, education and training, practice management and medicines management.
- **Experience of patients** covering the services provided, how they are provided and their involvement in local delivery plans.
- **Additional services**, e.g. contraception, maternity, cervical screening.

Why is data quality important? Full, accurate clinical records are essential for safe decision-making. They can highlight the health needs of a whole population and of specific groups, whilst forming a basis for justifying commissioning requirements. The nGMS links payment to recorded evidence of work done and – for the first time – to work not done but clinically justified, e.g. aspirin not being prescribed because of a contraindication. This latter approach is known as *exception coding*, which allows the practice to exclude from the process patients who are unsuitable or who do not consent to recommended clinical measures.

It is imperative that the correct READ codes are applied to the disease categories to enable the PCOs to gather the data they require on which to base the payments. These codes are readily available from the published literature. Codes should only be used when a disease has been fully investigated and diagnosed (e.g. use 'chest pain' *not* 'angina' until a positive exercise test has been performed). This will avoid patients going on to the disease register incorrectly.

How do you define data quality? Data is of high quality when it is:

Complete	all relevant information is included
Accurate	all information is correct and can be relied upon
Relevant	the information recorded has been agreed to be necessary and appropriate
Accessible	information is available at the point and time of need
Timely	information is kept up to date

Where to start. The use of READ codes in consultations, when compiling a note summary or entering data from laboratory results, Out of Hours services and secondary care is the only way that information can be easily entered and retrieved (it is not possible to search for information recorded in free text).

The use of templates and protocols ensures that all members of the team record the same information in a consistent fashion.

Practices need to agree what information should be included in note summaries and how new information coming into the practice via letters etc. is captured and recorded.

READ codes. READ codes are not intuitive. However, if you know what the first digit of a code stands for, you will be able to make choices between codes with a greater degree of certainty.

> Do be sure that you check the READ codes that are embedded in these as inappropriate codes will ensure that the entire team makes the same mistakes too

> Codes that begin with a NUMBER are classified as PROCESSES OF CARE
> Codes that begin with a CAPITAL LETTER are always DIAGNOSES
> Codes that begin with a LOWER-CASE LETTER are MEDICATIONS and APPLIANCES
> (EMIS uses its own drug codes that are mapped to READ)

READ codes are hierarchical. The more information you have, the greater the size of code (to a maximum of five digits). For example, G. . . . designates cardiovascular disease; G3 . . . is ischaemic heart disease and G33. . is angina pectoris. Practices should aim to record a useful level of clinical information. The software that will be used to identify what work practices have done and what to pay them 'Quality Management and Analysis System' – (QMAS) will use very specific codes. Practices should familiarise themselves with these codes and ensure that they are using them. They can be found on the DoH website but there are others that are more user-friendly, such as the EQUIP Section of the University of East Anglia.

Where to get help. All clinical systems contain a READ code dictionary, but this is often displayed in a limited and unhelpful way. The NHS Information Authority provides a free item of software called a Clinical Terminology Browser (TRISET), which is much better and is especially useful for non-clinical note summarisers.

The Primary Care Information Service (PRIMIS) exists specifically to help practices understand and improve their data quality. PRIMIS facilitators are employed by many PCOs and offer a free service to practices.

Many PCOs offer training in READ codes, exception coding and note summarisation.

Clinical system suppliers can offer help with templates and protocols.

The document 'Good Practice Guidelines for General Practice Electronic Patient Records' (version 3 September 2003) is an invaluable source of advice and guidance.

Enhancing practice/private income

Some diversification from core NHS work and opportunities to improve income may be:
- medico-legal examination and reporting;
- drug company research;
- occupational health;
- sports medicine;
- dispensing;
- Benefit Agency work;
- medical writing;
- PCO board work;
- out of hours for cooperatives;
- additional services for non-provider practices, e.g. family planning;
- enhanced services work for PCO initiatives, e.g. specialist clinics;
- medical work for hospital trusts; and
- medical education.

The level of pay varies enormously, with some of the most deserving being the least well remunerated!

Simon Cartwright (2003) in his book *Contract 2003 – A GPs Guide to Earning the Most* gives further examples of the private work of a GP as:
- acupuncture;
- authorship;
- committee fees;
- directorship, e.g. cooperative and ambulance trust;
- expert witness;
- hospice work;
- hospital work;
- independent tribunal service;
- medical audit advisory group work;
- medical research ethics committee;
- occupational health;
- pilot's licence;
- police surgeon;
- retainer, e.g. nursing homes/private schools/Ministry of Defence;
- review panel – disciplinary;
- sports medicine;
- summative assessment assessors;
- MRCGP examiner;
- travel clinic; and
- training/teaching.

Useful websites for *The practice*

Citizens Advice Bureau (CAB)	www.citizensadvice.org.uk/
Clinical Governance Bulletin	www.rsmpress.co.uk/cgb.htm
Clinical Governance Support Team	www.cgsupport.nhs.uk/
Clinical Terminology Browser	www.nhsia.nhs.uk/terms/pages
EQUIP	www.equip.nhs.uk
GMS Contract	www.doh.gov.uk/gmscontract/ infotech.htm
	www.nhsconfed.org/gmscontract
Good Practice Guidelines (GPC)	www.doh.gov.uk/gpepr/guidelines.pdf
Health Care Commission	*www.healthcarecommission.org.uk*
	www.cgsupport.org
National Institute of Clinical Excellence (NICE)	www.nice.org.uk
National Service Framework (NSF)	www.publications.doh.gov.uk/nsf/
NHS Modernisation Agency (NHSMA)	www.modern.nhs.uk
NHS Direct	www.nhsdirect.nhs.uk
NHS Pensions Agency	www.nhspa.gov.uk/index.cfm
NHS Walk-In Centres	www.nhs.uk/England/ noAppointmentNeeded/ walkinCentres/default.aspx
Out of Hours	www.out-of-hours.info/index.php? pid=10
Primary Care Information Services	www.primis.nhs.uk
QAMAS (Read Codes)	www.npfit.nhs.uk/programmes/qmas
Quality Outcomes Framework	www.doh.gov.uk/gmscontract/ qualityoutcomes.pdf
Prescription Pricing Authority (PPA)	www.ppa.nhs.uk
READ Codes	www.equip.ac.uk/readCodes/docs/ index.html
	www.acc.co.nz/for-providers/ resources/ read-code-database/
Royal College of General Practice (RCGP)	www.rcgp.org.uk
Royal College of Nursing (RCN)	www.rcn.org.uk

A full list of websites can be found on pages 192–197.

The patient

What patients want

Patients Concern is an organisation committed to promoting choice and empowerment for all health service users.

The following article has been reproduced by kind permission of the organisation:

It can be said that GPs are the friendly face of the medical profession. There are no white coats in the surgery and few bow ties. On the whole patients record a high level of satisfaction, with thoughtful surveys showing that the ability to communicate, knowledge of the patient and personal level of care are most likely to boost that satisfaction.

Every patient wants to be treated as an individual, not always an easy task for a doctor, as a succession of different people with different health care needs enter the surgery door. But when they can make the patient feel they really matter during those few minutes of a consultation, then the result will be trust in diagnosis and compliance with treatment.

The vast majority of complaints about GPs fielded by the *Patient Concern* help-line concern what is perceived as 'disrespect', often in forms that GPs might be astonished to hear. There are still doctors who use a large desk as a barrier, as though interviewing a junior employee, or who seldom raise their eyes from their computers to look at the person in front of them.

We can only feel that we are genuinely involved in our own care if our GP recognises that when we talk about our own body we are the experts. We can only retain autonomy if they acknowledge that when making health care choices we may have priorities and values that don't relate directly to the 'best' medical outcome. We need them to accept that they are imparting advice, not instruction, and that compromise may sometimes be necessary.

We always advise those lucky enough to have a choice of practice in their area to start by chatting to the receptionists, on the theory that empathetic doctors will employ empathetic staff. Dragons are more likely to be drawn to dragons. Of course, receptionists are the front line and have to exercise judgement in allocating doctors' valuable time. However, there is a widespread feeling that well-meaning staff may be affording doctors more protection than they need or want. Surely we should start from the presumption that we are all on the same side?

We hear frequent worries about access to medical records. Everyone knows that they can ask to see them, but most worry that this will 'upset' their doctors, that they will be labelled as problem patients – or even struck off. This may or may not be a justified fear but it does indicate an unsatisfied demand. One GP tells us that for the past 20 years he has encouraged his patients to read their notes as a matter of routine, and he has encountered neither litigation nor hysterical patients distressed by what they read. Sadly, he believes that he is unique. A routine check on notes, welcomed by the practice, could correct errors (audit shows that 40% of notes contain mistakes), prevent misunderstandings and promote co-operation.

There is a great deal more useful information that a visit to the surgery could provide us. A notice board listing details of all doctors at the practice (photos optional!) with qualifications, background and special interests is a welcome human touch. Most waiting rooms offer only the familiar rack of pamphlets on incontinence and prostate problems, which most visitors are too embarrassed to pick up. Some surgeries do better, offering a small library where we can investigate our condition further. If this is not possible, a list of reliable internet sites covering health matters would be valuable, and would not stretch the budget.

These days there is often a scattering of irritable notices about missed appointments and zero tolerance of rudeness to staff. So far I have never seen a notice explaining the functions and workings of the PCO – with an explanation of what out of hours cover is now available under their auspices – and seldom leaflets on the Patient Advice and Liaison Service (PALS) – see below. Vast numbers of patients have no idea of the existence of PCOs or PALS.

It remains to be seen how patients' views of GPs will change now that the cornerstone of the relationship – continuity of care – has been fundamentally changed by the nGMS. We shall now be registered with a practice rather than an individual doctor and GPs will observe office hours. No patient views were sought on these major changes.

Add this to the increasing number of practices that are now refusing to book appointments ahead, in order to conform to the 48 hour (now under review at the time of writing) making it more unlikely that we can see a doctor of our choice. All these changes seem to put us at arms length from our GPs. Walk in centres may beckon invitingly and it may take more effort and innovation to preserve that special family doctor relationship. (© Patient Concern. Contact by e-mail at patientconcern@hotmail.com).

The Patient Advice and Liaison Service (PALS) and your practice

PALS has recently been set up in every NHS Trust, in partnership with GP practices, as part of the government's 10-year plan to improve the services offered to patients and get the best out of the NHS. It aims to make the patient's journey through the NHS, including GP practices, as smooth as possible by actively listening to the views of patients, relatives, carers and visitors in making sure that suggestions, concerns and complaints are acted upon to continuously improve services.

There is now provision of 'on the spot' help in every PCO, with the power to negotiate immediate solutions or speedy resolutions of problems. PALS will listen and provide the relevant information and support to help resolve service users' concerns quickly and efficiently. They will liaise with staff and managers, and where appropriate, with other PALS services as well as health and related organisations, to facilitate a resolution. PALS will also act as a gateway to appropriate independent advice and advocacy support from local and national sources, including Independent Complaints Advocacy Services (ICAS). PALS staffs are well-briefed on links to organisations able to facilitate provision of appropriate advice and support.

PALS provide accurate information to patients, carers and families, about the PCO's services (as well as other health-related issues), using accredited and reliable sources, thus acting as a catalyst for change and improvement. They will be an early warning system for the PCO and also a key source of information and feedback. The PALS service monitors problems and proactively seeks patients' experience of health care, including problems arising, and highlights gaps in services by:

- Developing and maintaining an information resource capable of collating and analysing all issues dealt with by PALS.
- Providing information, advice and training on their service and issues raised by service users to staff.
- PALS should submit regular anonymised reports to the PCO board, and also liaise with service managers, directorates and the board on policy issues that involve PALS and customer care/service user issues.
- Establishing and maintaining clear formal routes for feeding back emerging themes to clinical governance and quality, and to individual departments.

PALS operates within a local network with other PALS in their area and work across organisational boundaries (e.g. GP practices and PCOs) to ensure a seamless service for patients who move between (and use different parts of) the NHS for the care they need. In this way they will ensure that patients' concerns are picked up and dealt with in the most appropriate way for the person concerned.

The PALS national free phone number is

0800 389 7671 (24 hours).

Gaining patient feedback

Most GPs have long been aware that one of the secrets of successful general practice is to realise 'it ain't what you do but the way that you do it'.

The public has often judged doctors on this as 'their bedside manner' and GPs have researched and written on this as the 'human factor' (Dixon *et al.* 1999). Now the GMC includes evidence of relationships with patients as one of the attributes of a good doctor, and objective evidence of this is required for appraisal and will be required for revalidation in future.

The nGMS also rewards practices for undertaking patients surveys and acting on them. Thus, every GP will need in future to capture evidence of their interaction with patients and build this into their personal development plan and appraisal.

How to gain feedback

Patient surveys are the best way of capturing systematic evidence in this field. They can give both quantitative and qualitative feedback and are simple and easy to administer in general practice. Results can be presented back to the participating clinician in a form that is easy to understand and can compare performance against benchmarks for their peers on a local or national basis.

In order to satisfy appraisal and revalidation however, something more than the basic practice level survey sufficient for GMS2 is needed as GPs will need individual-level feedback on their own performance. This level of data can be provided both by the Improving Practice Questionnaire (IPQ) and General Practice Assessment Questionnaire (GPAQ) approved for GMS2 and by the Doctors' Interpersonal Skills Questionnaire (DISQ) for locums and sessional doctors who work in different sites.

It is likely that external analysis of these results will be required for revalidation to ensure probity and to preserve confidentiality. A minimum of 40 questionnaires per GP is vital to achieve statistical power from the feedback and avoid skewing of results by individuals (Wensing *et al.* 1997).

Other forms of patient feedback are also important. These may include individual testimonies, complaints and documented practice achievements. These will clearly be more valid than receiving "thank you" notes in christmas cards although we always like to receive the latter! Such feedback should be included in a file and discussed with an appraiser. It must be remembered that patients are highly reluctant to make negative individual comments about GPs and when they do, the reasons prompting this should at least demand reflection and analysis.

What sort of survey?

For gaining feedback on an individual's relationships with patients, an exit survey where the patient completes a questionnaire shortly after seeing a doctor is most effective. Response rates are higher than those in postal surveys, and only those patients who have seen that doctor recently are surveyed. Postal surveys, unless specifically targeted at recent users, tend to reach infrequent or irregular users and their feedback may not be based on contemporary experience and may be open to 'inoculation' from other patients or the media. Exit surveys are simpler and cheaper to administer.

Receiving the results of patient feedback

Do not underestimate the power of this and the emotions it can induce, especially if the results are below average. Usually the results will have been processed externally and presented in an easy-to-read form with benchmarks and scales for each question. A breakdown of results relative to the age and gender of patient surveyed and whether they are seeing their usual doctor or not is often also provided, which can produce dramatic variances.

Results should be given confidentially to each doctor but it is always best to agree on someone in advance with whom the results can be shared. This can be a colleague, appraiser, friend or spouse but is vital to allow you to express and share the emotions the feedback can elicit. Most GPs are highly conscientious and feedback usually elicits a strong desire to improve further even with above average scores.

It is also rare to get a totally negative score and as scores are given against each question, the method of identifying strengths first and then potential weaknesses can be used when discussing the feedback with colleagues.

After a while GPs will often feel comfortable sharing their results with their peers and practice manager, which can be useful for team planning, but there is a need to be sensitive to those with lower scores who may feel threatened by this approach.

Personal development planning

Once GPs have received the results of their feedback it is vital to use this to improve practice and make a difference. Each and every doctor should be able to find something to address in their results and if they are near perfect then they could be very useful educators and resources to those who do not score so well.

Patient feedback though is only one important element in a GP's portfolio of skill-technical competence, relationships with peers, probity, availability and acquisition of new knowledge and skills are all vital elements too. Patient feedback should be appraised besides these other factors to give a holistic view of an individual's performance.

With the help of a mentor or appraiser, skill development to address the results of feedback can be identified and planned. There is evidence that structured communication-skills workshops can result in a significant improvement in doctors subsequent survey ratings – even after one day (Greco *et al.* 1998). Shadowing or observing other colleagues or learning basic consultation skills can also bring about significant improvements in practice and can even help with time management (Beck *et al.* 2002). All this needs to be recorded so that it can later be presented as evidence for revalidation.

> So it is probably possible to be brilliant with patients yet still be a poor GP overall, but it is virtually impossible to be a good overall GP without being good with patients!

Practice and team planning

Where practices are mature enough it can be really useful to share the relative strengths and weaknesses of the whole team as part of a practice development plan. No individual GP is likely to be good at everything but it is important for patients to be able to access and choose a doctor or nurse with the attributes they need. This collated overview of feedback can also help explain why some doctors seem more popular than others and have longer waiting times for their services.

Why good relationships are important

Regular sampling of patient experience and perception of clinician's communication skills is rightly seen as a priority by the GMC, government and PCOs.

There is a range of evidence showing that good relationships help reduce complaints, improve compliance with treatment and increase job satisfaction (Stewart 1995). In the new era of patient choice, a doctor's manner may be the crucial factor in the success of a health care-related business or practice when competition becomes a reality.

As my old GP trainer said to me on my first day as a GP registrar 'you can be struck off for three things, adultery, addiction and association (e.g. with an unqualified midwife)'.

The IPQ form at the end of this chapter has been used in over 60 PCOs across the United Kingdom, involving over 200,000 patients. The IPQ is also being used for appraisals and future revalidation as a way in which clinicians can gather evidence about their relationships with patients. The IPQ is approved by the RCN's accreditation unit, and participants are awarded eight continuing education points.

> Patients will judge you on three things:
> *   affability,
> *   availability, and
> *   ability, and *in that order*!

Using complaints to improve practice

Nobody likes to receive complaints about their practice. They are time-consuming and often cause a lot of heartache amongst the team. In addition to PALS discussed earlier, each practice should have its own practice-based complaints procedure. Most complaints can be resolved in-house but some may go further and even involve litigation or the use of the formal NHS complaint procedures (2004).

The aim of a practice-based complaints procedure should be to satisfy the needs of the complainants. Often this may only need an adequate explanation and apology where appropriate, whilst being fair to all concerned. Honesty, courtesy and sympathy in the handling of a complaint will often go a long way towards defusing a potentially difficult situation.

Dealing with complaints

Practices have a duty to deal with complaints quickly and sensitively whilst keeping written records of all contacts with patients. Patients must also be made aware of their rights to take their complaint to the relevant PCO. Written information about the complaints procedure should be available to patients in the surgery.

Each practice should have a nominated PHCT member and GP to deal with complaints. Meticulous record keeping is of paramount importance. Copies of letters must be kept, and notes, dates and times of all telephone conversations should be logged.

If a patient complains in person, say at reception, then the receptionist should offer an immediate meeting with a member of staff in private, so that the complaint can be recorded on an in-house complaint form. This should be completed, dated, timed and signed by the patient and the member of staff. The patient can be given information about the complaints procedure there and then.

All complaints should be reviewed regularly as this may enable the PHCT to identify deficiencies within the practice, both clinical and non-clinical, which if addressed promptly and honestly can improve the quality of the service that you can provide. Analysis of complaints fits in well with the process of significant-event auditing, further details of which can be found on page 114.

Learning from complaints

Complaints to the practice can be a valuable tool to look at your practice, how it works and how staff performs within the team. Anecdotal evidence suggests that complaints seem to involve mainly appointment systems, telephone answering delays, prescriptions and staff attitudes as the major grievances. Medical Defence Union (MDU) research showed that commonest reasons for complaints to be made about GPs in 2001 and 2002 were failure or delayed referral, medication errors, failure or delayed visit, failure to perform or inadequate examination, and attitude/rudeness.

New NHS complaint procedure (2004)

The practice should be aware that complaint procedure changes came into force on 30 July 2004 as the following article reproduced by kind permission of the MDU, by Dr Paul Colbrook, a MDU medico-legal adviser, explains:

> Regulations have been laid before Parliament to enable the Healthcare Commission (the Commission) to operate the revised independent review stage of the NHS complaints procedure. The Commission began to receive requests for review of complaints in July 2004 and the regulations came into force on 30 July 2004.
>
> The changes to independent review mark the beginning of what is likely to be a comprehensive shake-up of the NHS complaints procedure which has been left largely unchanged since its introduction in 1996.

The first stage of the complaints procedure – local resolution – is currently under review by the Department of Health and is likely to change sometime in 2005. The third stage, referral to the ombudsman, remains unchanged and complaints can be referred to the ombudsman at any stage.

The changes apply only to England. There are different procedures for Scotland, Wales and Northern Ireland (© The MDU (2004). All rights reserved).

Independent review

One of the MDU's criticisms of the previous independent review procedures was that they varied greatly in the quality of their recommendations and the hearings could be very adversarial. The changes are designed to make independent review more consistent and less adversarial for all parties involved. Medical defence organisations will be provided with specific guidance but, in the meantime, this chapter sets out the way in which the new procedure is likely to operate, based on the MDU's understanding of the regulations and on discussions with the Commission. Doctors subject to the new independent review procedures are advised to seek advice from their medical defence organisation.

Three stages

There are three stages to the new independent review system: review, investigation and panel hearings. Patients or their representatives can ask the Commission to review a complaint if they are not satisfied with the result of local resolution, if local resolution has not been completed within 6 months or if a complaints manager has decided not to investigate a complaint because it was outside the time limits.

The Commission will review all complaints it receives. It may decide to investigate the complaint further, and as a result of that investigation a panel may be held. Everyone who asks for a complaint to be reviewed by the Commission will get a review but there is no automatic right to an investigation. The Commission expects to receive 5000 review requests annually and to conduct between 800 and 900 investigations.

The request for a review may be made orally or in writing (including electronically) either direct to the Commission or to the subject of the complaint. The request must be made within 2 months of the date on which the complainant receives the local resolution response.

Decisions

The regulations do not contain a timetable for independent review, but the Commission has set its own limits that may change. For example, the Commission aims to acknowledge receipt of a complaint within 2 days, ask for a response from the organisation complained about within 20 days and have a decision on whether an investigation is warranted within 10 days. The Commission currently expects the whole procedure to take between 5 and 6 months.

The Commission has a wide-ranging number of decisions about the complaint open to it. One major change is that the Commission can look at different aspects of treatment, provided by different health care practitioners, and it can reach different decisions in relation to different parts of the complaint. The decisions open to it are:
• Take no further action.

- Refer the complaint back to the GP, NHS Trust or PCO with recommendations about what can be done to resolve it.
- Investigate the complaint further before deciding whether to refer to a panel.
- Refer the complaint to a panel, with the agreement of the complainant.
- Refer the complaint to the appropriate professional regulator, e.g. GMC.
- Refer the complaint to a local authority.
- Refer the complaint to the Health Service Ombudsman.
- Consider the complaint as part of, or in conjunction with, any other investigation it is conducting as part of the exercise of its other functions.

Investigation

If the Commission decides to investigate the complaint further, it will notify those involved of its proposed terms of reference within 10 working days of the date it notified them of the investigation. There are 10 working days in which to make any comments to the Commission.

In order to investigate the complaint properly, the Commission may request any person or body to produce information or documents it considers necessary. It will make these requests in writing and specify the information requested and why it is relevant. It will not make a request for information which is confidential and relates to a living person unless the person has consented or the information is anonymised.

Panels

Panels will be made up of independent lay members, and health care professionals may not be panel members. The Commission may reach a decision based on its own investigation, rather than convening a panel. However, at the investigation stage, if a complainant or the doctor complained against requests for a review panel, the Commission must arrange for the complaint to be considered by a panel of three people.

A panel, where established, must allow participants to be heard in person and ensure they are kept informed about proceedings, including the composition of the panel, the time and date of the hearing and the names of those to be interviewed or from whom it proposes to take advice or evidence.

Participants may be accompanied or represented by a friend or advocate, including a medico-legal adviser, though they may only act as supporters.

Report from Commission's investigations

The Commission must prepare a written report of an investigation as soon as is reasonably practicable. The report will summarise the nature of the complaint, the Commission's findings and make recommendations for resolving the complaint. It may also suggest ways of improving the service complained about.

The final report will be sent to:
- The complainant together with a letter explaining the right to refer the complaint to the Health Service Ombudsman.
- The subject of the complaint.
- In the case of a complaint involving a primary care provider, to the relevant PCO.
- Any relevant strategic health authority.
- An anonymised version of the report will be posted on the Commission's website.

GPs will be responsible for implementing recommendations relating to them that come out of a case review or panel hearing and will be expected to be able to demonstrate how systems have improved. Strategic health authorities will be asked to follow up recommendations routinely. Failure to implement recommendations may result in further action by the Commission.

The outline of the procedure above is the best information the MDU had at the time of writing this chapter in July 2004. Our medico-legal advisers are always happy to answer members' questions about the new procedures.

Useful websites for *The patient*

Client-Focused Evaluations Program (CFEP)	www.latix.ex.ac.uk/cfedp www.ex.ac.uk/cfep
Commission for Patient and Public Involvement in Health (CPPIH)	www.cppih.org/index.html
Health Care Commission	www.healthcarecommission.org.uk
Health Service Ombudsman	http://www.ombudsman.org.uk/hse/
Independent Complaints Advocacy Services (ICAS)	www.dh.gov.uk
Medical Defence Union (MDU)	www.the-mdu.com/
Medical Protection Society	www.mps.org.uk
National Association of Patient Participation	http://www.napp.org.uk/
NHS Complaints Procedure	http://www.nhs.uk/england/ aboutTheNHS/complainCompliment.cmsx
NHS Patient Survey Programme Advice Centre	www.nhssurveys.org
Patient Advice and Liaison Service (PALS)	www.nelh.nhs.uk/pals/ www.dh.gov.uk
Patient Association	www.patients-association.com
Patient Concern	www.patientconcern.org.uk
Patient Support Groups	www.patient.co.uk
Shipman Enquiry	www.the-shipman-inquiry.org.uk

A full list of websites can be found on pages 192–197.

IMPROVING PRACTICE QUESTIONNAIRE

DOCTOR'S NAME:

YOU CAN HELP THIS GENERAL PRACTICE IMPROVE ITS SERVICE

.   The practice and the doctors at this surgery would welcome your honest feedback.

.   Please do not write your name on this survey.

.   Please read and complete this survey **after** you have seen the doctor.

PLEASE RATE EACH OF THE FOLLOWING AREAS BY <u>CIRCLING</u> ONE NUMBER ON EACH LINE.

	Poor	Fair	Good	Very Good	Excellent
ABOUT THE PRACTICE					
1. Your level of satisfaction with the practice's opening hours	1	2	3	4	5
2. Ease of contacting the practice on the telephone	1	2	3	4	5
3. Satisfaction with the day and time arranged for your appointment	1		3	4	5
4. Chances of seeing a doctor within 48 hours	1		3	4	5
5. Chances of seeing the doctor of <u>your</u> choice	1	2	3	4	5
6. Opportunity of speaking to a doctor on the telephone when necessary	1	2	3	4	5
7. Comfort level of waiting room (eg. chairs, magazines)	1	2	3	4	5
8. Length of time waiting in the practice to see the doctor	1	2	3	4	5
ABOUT THE DOCTOR *(whom you just saw)*					
9. My overall satisfaction with this visit to the doctor	1	2	3	4	5
10. The warmth of the doctor's greeting to me was	1	2	3	4	5
11. On this visit I would rate the doctor's ability to really listen to me as	1	2	3	4	5
12. The doctor's explanations of things to me were	1	2	3	4	5
13. The extent to which I felt reassured by this doctor was	1	2	3	4	5
14. My confidence in this doctor's ability is	1	2	3	4	5
15. The opportunity the doctor gave me to express my concerns or fears was	1	2	3	4	5
16. The respect shown to me by this doctor was	1	2	3	4	5

PLEASE TURN OVER

ABOUT THE DOCTOR (Continued....)	Poor	Fair	Good	Very Good	Excellent
17. The amount of time given to me for this visit was	1	2	3	4	5
18. This doctor's consideration of my personal situation in deciding a treatment or advising me was	1	2	3	4	5
19. The doctor's concern for me as a person in this visit was	1	2	3	4	5
20. The recommendation I would give to my friends about this doctor would be	1	2	3	4	5

ABOUT THE STAFF

	Poor	Fair	Good	Very Good	Excellent
21. The manner in which you are treated by the reception staff	1		3	4	5
22. Respect shown for your privacy and confidentiality		2	3	4	5
23. Information provided by the practice about its services (eg. repeat prescriptions, test results, cost of private certificates)		2	3	4	5
24. The opportunity for making compliments or complaints to the practice about its service and quality of care		2	3	4	5

FINALLY

	Poor	Fair	Good	Very Good	Excellent
25. The information provided by this practice about how to prevent illness and stay healthy (eg. alcohol use, health risk of smoking, diet habits, etc) was	1	2	3	4	5
26. The availability and administration of reminder systems for ongoing health checks is	1	2	3	4	5
27. The practice's respect of your right to seek a second opinion or complementary medicine was..	1	2	3	4	5

Any comments about how this <u>practice</u> could improve their service?_____

_____

_____

Any comments about how the <u>doctor</u> could improve?_____

_____

_____

The following questions provide us only with general information about the range of people who have responded to this survey. This information will **not** be used to identify you and will remain confidential.

How old are you, in years? _____   What is your postcode? _____

Are you ☐ Female   Was this visit with your usual GP? ☐ Yes

☐ Male   ☐ No

How many years have you been attending this Practice? ☐ Less than five years

☐ Five to ten years

☐ More than ten years

THANK YOU FOR YOUR TIME AND ASSISTANCE

The primary health care team

The GP's perspective – counting the 'beans'

To be an effective GP you need to be a team player. Gone are the days when a GP was able to work in glorious isolation, perhaps supported by a receptionist and a part-time nurse. Perhaps this still applies to most doctors worldwide, but the NHS has changed all that for those of us in the UK.

General practice is now an extremely complex business. We work for a micromanaged and closely regulated organisation and are all accountable to our patients, our PCOs, the NHS and the GMC, to name but a few! We need to pass examinations and be admitted to the primary medical performers list. To remain on the list we need to have an annual appraisal and be revalidated every 5 years. We work in a target-driven environment and our very livelihood depends upon achieving QOF points and submitting paperwork, plans and audits on anything ranging from courses in Health and Safety at Work and Control of Substances Hazardous to Health (COSHH) courses.

Obviously we cannot do all this on our own. To be a happy, contented and successful GP, not to mention making sufficient money to support our chosen lifestyles, we need to be supported by a happy, contented, well-paid, knowledgeable and skilled PHCT. This team may include partners, sessional GPs, GP registrars, nurse practitioners, practice nurses, health visitors, community nurses, managers, audit clerks, counsellors, health care assistants, receptionists and dispensers.

No longer is it sufficient for patient services to be provided with a brief record of the consultation annotated in their notes. Now everything must be recorded in the right place and in the right format. We must audit what we have done and then provide the same service at intervals and keep auditing it forever. Somehow we need to be able to motivate our teams to maintain the right mindset and to ensure that they are able to do this at each and every patient encounter.

A practice may offer a huge variety and choice of services from chiropody to echocardiography, but at the end of the day, they still need to be able to provide basic medical services to their local community. Patients will continue to present with undifferentiated medical problems and symptoms which may be a minor self-limiting illness, but could contain a clue about some more serious underlying pathology. Patients will still need home visits, for instance the elderly housebound with chronic disease and palliative care. They will still need cervical cytology and monitoring of their chronic disease. There will still be children at risk in our communities who have a record of multiple consultations and parents and carers who are known to the practice. Although there are no NSFs or QOFs on offer, our patients will still have Parkinson's disease, multiple sclerosis, psoriasis and rheumatoid arthritis.

Ultimately we will be judged as a PHCT on those aspects of our care that cannot be measured easily, as well as those that can be.

Our clinical knowledge can be measured by examinations. Our best behaviour, consultation skills, can be assessed using a video or a simulated surgery. Specific clinical outcomes are now measured and remunerated by the nGMS. Perhaps, care, kindness, empathy, rapport, dedication and sense of humour can be measured by levels of patient's satisfaction, but is this a main drive for change within the new NHS?

GPs still like to think that they are the leaders and focus of their PHCT. Often they will own the business but are they up to the challenge of:

- working at the 'coalface';
- maintaining their knowledge and skills;
- motivating and leading their PHCT;
- being well respected and giving confidence to their patients;
- meeting all the PCO and new contract targets;
- being a profitable organisation;
- promoting and being committed to the values of best GP, year on year, in good times and bad; and
- having the ability to understand and identify with our patients and our communities.

Patients are now offered a choice of who they can see and to choose the most suitable form of consultation to meet their individual needs. Choices include:

- Telephone triage by a nurse or a doctor
- Telephone consultation with a nurse or a doctor
- Emergency face-to-face consultation with a nurse or a doctor
- Booked face-to-face consultation with a nurse or a doctor
- Face-to-face consultation with a health care assistant for venepuncture, blood pressure measurement or checking weight

Patients can phone NHSDirect, attend a Walk-In Centre, a Minor Injuries Unit, or perhaps an Accident and Emergency Department. Shortly, they will be able to register with more than one practice, one near their work and another where they live. GPs no longer have a monopoly on front line primary care. The nGMS allows GPs to opt out of certain 'non-core' activities, such as minor surgery, child health surveillance, and family planning. Other providers such as BUPA or Prime Care are entering the marketplace and are bidding to provide medical services including out of hours. Contracts are provided not only on the basis of quality, but also on cost. Traditional general practice is long gone.

To survive, practices need to be:

- open to change;
- innovative;
- efficient;
- well managed;
- popular and respected in their community; and
- multi-skilled.

Most importantly, GPs need to be kind, caring and sensitive individuals. They need to take a holistic approach to health care. To survive in the new NHS, 'bean' counting will become increasingly important. It is hoped that this second edition of the workbook will not only help you count the 'beans' but remind you that there are perhaps more important things than bean counting, in being a good doctor and leader.

Leadership

In addition to undertaking one of the most rewarding but demanding professions you have, by electing to be a GP, also entered one of the most complex

- How do you measure care and empathy?
- Do you make enough of your time available, and are you flexible?
- Are you prepared to make that extra home visit, after 6.30 p.m. or at weekends when you are not on duty?
- Do you give the families of your terminal care patients, or indeed any other patients in distress, your mobile and home telephone numbers?
- Do you have the capacity and skill to build rapport?
- Are you able to communicate and do you have a shared vision about providing care to your patients within your PHCT?

areas of British life, the 'small business'. In some respects small business is similar to any group undertaking in that the outcome is directly proportional to the vision, input and guidance of the leader – hence the term *leadership*.

Leadership is a dynamic process that deserves study. Though this is a massive area and this chapter does not make an attempt to deal with all aspects of the topic, a Google search will normally result in more than 4.5 million sites to help you.

Leadership is a relational process involving interactions between leaders, team members and sometimes outside agencies, e.g. PCO. It is a quality and skill that is both admired and needed in our society, and one that offers huge potential rewards. Do not confuse leadership with popularity, as being popular is an added bonus but it certainly is not as important as being fair, consistent and open in all your dealings with staff and partners alike. Lead by example and few people will fail to follow.

So how do you develop your own leadership skills? You have to start somewhere so consider the following:

1   Set and maintain high personal standards, for example:
    • Your commitment to your work
    • Your appearance
    • Your timekeeping.
2   Get to know your staff, their abilities, their aspirations and where they best fit into the team – which might not be where they are now!
3   How can you change or improve their working lives?

The first item above is something that you are best able to control once you have appreciated its importance and despite the many changes in general practice you still enjoy a profession with considerable status. Patients will look up to you for an example, so just as it is difficult for a heavily overweight doctor to credibly give advice on the importance of losing weight, similarly you could encounter problems counselling a member of staff for poor timekeeping if you are frequently late for work. Similarly, however much you strive to be 'one of the team' your opinions as a GP will always carry considerable weight within primary care, and considerable status within the community as a whole.

Getting to know your staff takes time and effort. As with most topics in this workbook, it should be done with the prior knowledge and approval of your partners; there will normally be a partner who has specific responsibility for staff and they should be able to provide background information in addition to that you already have.

The third item above is more complex and you have limited resources. However, one constantly underfunded area is the non-clinical staff-training budget. This is one area where you might be able to make a difference.

The following will help in the process:

1   Speak to your business/practice manager and explain what you wish to do and achieve. They will be able to provide much of the information, advise you when appraisals were last completed and show you the PDP of each staff member where appropriate.
2   Ask your manager for a copy of each person's job specification and last two appraisals. To avoid too much bulk, consider asking for this information electronically.
3   Ask your manager what funding arrangements exist for non-clinical staff training if you are not already aware. Ask about the NHS

Individual Learning Accounts (ILAs) including the uptake in the last 2 years.

4 Agree with the manager about a series of individual meetings with staff as there may be considerable advantages in the manager attending or becoming actively involved in such meetings. Be realistic in your planning, and depending on the number of staff one interview per month may well be all that you can achieve.

5 Carry out the above-mentioned meetings, ensuring that staff know why they are being 'interviewed'. Remember the importance of indirect questions (by using what? when? where? why? who?), as you are after all the master of such discussions. Think what you can extract from a patient in just a few minutes!

Challenges in probity

An essential feature of good leadership is that it raises the issue of probity and intellectual honesty. This is one of the areas to be recorded in your NHS appraisal form. This includes:

1 What safeguards are in place to ensure propriety in your financial and commercial affairs, research work, use of professional position, etc.? Have there been any problems?

2 What factors in your workplace, or externally, constrain you in this area?

Probity is about honesty and personal integrity. Of course, money, accounting and what you do with cash fees are important as is intellectual honesty. This raises questions about how you record a blood pressure of 151/91, when the target to gain valuable QOF points is 149/89.

There is a potentially exhaustive list of situations where there are opportunities for our honesty and personal integrity to become compromised.

For example, have you ever thought about a consultant working privately, who perhaps suggests a surgical procedure that cannot be wholly justified on the evidence of benefit against risk or perhaps they continue with clinical reviews over an inappropriately long period.

Before completing the probity section of your next NHS appraisal, perhaps you can consider the following:

- Do I use an accountant to audit my professional and personal accounts?
- Do I have a system to ensure that my expense claims are correct?
- Do I always pay cash fees into the Partnership Account?
- Have I ever received a gift, disproportionate to the service provided?
- Has pharmaceutical entertainment or a gift ever influenced my prescribing?
- Are my medical records always factually correct?
- Have I ever changed a physiological measurement to meet a clinical target?
- What systems do I have in place to monitor my professional and financial activities?
- Do I work within a supportive peer group structure?
- Do I have a 'buddy system' and encourage a professional colleague to review my clinical work and research?

- Is your prescribing ever influenced by a drug company sponsored dinner?
- Do you work in a single-handed practice, or in a partnership, where there will be more opportunities to monitor your professional and financial affairs?
- Do you undertake a significant amount of unsupervised private medical work?
- Do you undertake pharmaceutical sponsored research?

- Can you ever see yourself being challenged?
- If so, how do you manage these personal and professional dilemmas?

The practice nurses' perspective

The role of the practice nurse is critical in delivering key clinical quality elements of the nGMS. Developments in primary care provide front-line nurses with opportunities to work in different and new ways. This includes expansion of the role in chronic disease management, minor illness, and first contact care and minor surgery. Nurses are therefore able to play an important part in helping a practice to expand services, to reach more patients and meet targets. In order to achieve this vision, nurses will need to be competent and confident in taking on these new roles. They will need to be supported and trained and have access to professional advice and CPD.

Services provided by Practice Nurses will continue to develop, expand and extend. In order to deliver high quality care the local community PHCTs will need to include trained ancillary staff and specialist practice nurses. As such, primary care nursing will need effective leadership if it is to take on new roles, work differently and deliver the improvements for patients and communities. This requires greater understanding of team development and management capability.

Practice nurses already undertake a range of roles and responsibilities. These vary considerably from practice to practice, in both levels of decision-making and autonomous clinical responsibility. The range of work that practice nurses perform is becoming broader as more nurses take on systematic care of chronic diseases and the triaging of minor illness and may well include:

- treatment room sessions;
- chronic disease management;
- home visiting;
- new patient checks;
- well person clinics;
- primary prevention and health promotion work;
- travel health;
- vaccination clinics;
- anti-coagulation clinics; and
- asthma, diabetes, coronary heart disease, chronic obstructive pulmonary disease and hypertension clinics.

Developments in practice nursing

The DoH document 'Liberating the Talents' (DoH 2002c) identified three core functions provided by nurses in primary care, irrespective of their title, employer or setting:

1 First contact/acute assessment, diagnosis, care, treatment and referral
2 Continuing care, rehabilitation, chronic disease management and delivering NSFs
3 Public health/health protection and promotion programmes that improve health and reduce inequalities

'Liberating the Talents' also describes a new three-part framework for nursing in primary care:

1 *Planning services in a new way* – provision of services based on an assessment of need, not who should do what or the enthusiasm of a particular profession. Patients and communities should be involved in service changes and provided with greater choice and a greater voice.
2 *Developing clinical roles* – setting up new services and changing existing ones. There will be more generalists working in teams. Support workers and health care assistants will become a more important part of the PHCT. More nurses will develop advanced and specialist skills to support generalists. There will be greater collaboration between health, social

care, hospitals, community care and primary care. Less emphasis will be put on protecting professional roles with the development of joint posts.

3 *Securing better care* – improving the working environment in which front-line staff work. All nurses, wherever employed, should have access to clinical supervision, professional advice, continuing professional development, good IT support and the knowledge and skills they need to provide high-quality care that is based on sound evidence.

The Chief Nursing Officer presented 10 key roles for nurses in the document 'Making a difference: strengthening the nursing, midwifery and health visiting contribution to health and healthcare' (DoH 1999). These were reinforced in 'The NHS Plan' and the 'Liberating the Talents' documents as follows:

- To order diagnostic investigations such as pathology tests and X-rays
- To make and receive referrals direct, say, to and from a therapist or pain consultant
- To admit and discharge patients for specific conditions within agreed protocols
- To manage patient case loads, say, for diabetes or rheumatology
- To run clinics, say, for ophthalmology or dermatology
- To prescribe medicines and treatments
- To carry out a wide range of resuscitation procedures including defibrillation
- To perform minor surgery and outpatient procedures
- To triage patients using the latest IT to the most appropriate health professional
- To take a lead in the way local health services are organised and the way that they are run

Nurse prescribing

Qualified district nurses and health visitors are able to prescribe from the nurses' formulary which includes wound care products, continence aids and other products used by community nurses in their care for patients. Prescribing rights are now extended to practice nurses. The new Extended Formulary with Supplementary prescribing both provide a more extensive list of prescription only medicines that can be used for specific medical conditions.

In terms of the Supplementary prescribing above, nurses can prescribe a wider range of prescription only medicines, within the limits of their competencies. This requires the consent of the patient, and written authorisation from the GP which is reviewed on an annual basis.

It is for PCOs and SHAs to consider, in the light of local priorities, which nurses in their areas should undertake training for prescribing.

Developing new roles in practice requires careful planning. The Exploring New Roles in Practice project (ENRiP) produced a user-friendly, evidence-based guide covering the main issues to be considered when developing new roles. Part one presents the key issues in the form of questions in seven sections, including management issues, professional issues, resource issues and effectiveness and outcomes. Part two picks up on these questions and discusses them further. The document 'Developing key roles for nurses and midwives: a guide for managers' (DoH 2002a) provides a full description of professional and legal aspects of extending the role of the nurse.

Professional development for practice nurses

As registered nurses, practice nurses are personally accountable for their practice. The Nursing and Midwifery Council (NMC) is charged, through an Act of Parliament, to maintain the standards of the profession. The Code of Professional Conduct (NMC 2002) issued by the NMC is a binding document to which nurses must adhere.

> To practice competently, registered nurses must possess the knowledge, skills and abilities required for lawful, safe and effective practice without direct supervision. The nurse must acknowledge the limits of her/his professional competence and only undertake practice and accept responsibilities for those activities in which they are competent. (para 6.2)

Practice nurses will require good employment conditions that include appraisals, clinical supervision and professional advice. They will also require access to CPD. Their employment conditions should take into account that for CPD to be effective, it should be taken in paid working time with backfill costs from their employers.

This workbook seeks to not only assist in the identification of CPD needs, but also identify opportunities for development that will lead to improved quality of patient care.

Useful websites for *The primary health care team*

Association of Independent Specialist Medical Accountants	http://www.aisma.org.uk/about.asp
Association of Managers in General Practice	www.ihm.org.uk
Association of Medical Secretaries, Practice Managers, Administrators and Receptionists (AMSPAR)	www.amspar.co.uk/frameset.htm
British Nursing Association	www.bna.co.uk
Control of Substance Hazardous to Health Regulations 2002 (COSHH)	www.hse.gov.uk/hthdir/noframes/coshh
Exploring New Roles in Practice (ENRiP)	www.shef.ac.uk/snm/research/enrip/
General Medical Council (GMC)	www.gmc-uk.org
General Practice Finance Corporation	www.gpfc.co.uk/
Institute of Health Service Managers	www.ihm.org.uk/
Liberating the Talents	www.dh.gov.uk/assetRoot/04/07/62/50/04076250.pdf
Medical Management Services	www.medman.co.uk/pcn/index.htm
National Association of Sessional GPs NASGP *(formerly known as the National Association of Non Principals – NANP)*	www.nasgp.org.uk
National Counselling Service for Sick Doctors	http://www.ncssd.org.uk/
NHSDirect	www.nhsdirect.nhs.uk

NHS Individual Learning Accounts	www.dh.gov.uk/PolicyAndGuidance/ HumanResourcesAndTraining/ LearningAndPersonal Development/
NHS Plan	www.dh.gov.uk
Nurse Prescribing	www.doh.gov.uk/nurseprescribing
Nursing and Midwifery Council (NMC)	www.nmc-uk.org
Royal College of General Practice (RCGP)	www.rcgp.org.uk
Royal College of Nursing (RCN)	www.rcn.org.uk
School of Health and Related Research – University of Sheffield (ScHARR)	www.shef.ac.uk
The Wisdom Centre – Education and Training for the NHS	www.wisdomnet.co.uk/default.asp

A full list of websites can be found on pages 192–197.

PART 2

Where do we start

The practice professional development plan

The practice professional development plan (PPDP)

In the past, GP and practice education has tended to be haphazard, often shaped by other people's perceptions of our needs. This method is refreshingly different, putting you and your practice at the centre of the learning process. The aim of this workbook is to enable you to identify your learning and development priorities. It also deals with how to collect the evidence of learning and discusses the use of portfolios in learning.

For education and learning to be effective it needs to be appropriate, both for our patients and us. At the heart of the PPDP is the assessment of both of these elements. No two practices are the same and every practice plan will be subtly, or dramatically, different from another's. It may be appropriate to build into this plan the needs of the PCO.

To start with, a practice will need to assess the health needs of its patients (this sounds more daunting than it really is). It will need to involve the whole team in looking at individuals' strengths, weaknesses and learning styles. Subsequently, it can identify its development priorities, which can be considered alongside the health needs of its patients.

This workbook provides a step-by-step guide to achieving and recording a development plan uniquely tailored to your needs and the needs of your practice. It will help you to work out your aims and objectives over the following years, as well as how and when you plan to achieve them.

This development plan needs to be owned jointly by the members of the practice and not imposed by one individual. To ensure success, members of the team will need to feel that they have contributed to the PPDP and that it belongs to them and should include sessional doctors and other staff.

The personal development plan (PDP)

When you take the decision to develop your own PDP, begin by writing down your aims and objectives.
- What do you want to achieve over the next 5 years?
- Which specific actions need to be done to achieve it?
- How and when are these specific actions going to be tackled?

This workbook illustrates a number of methods by which learning needs can be identified. An important theme that emerges is the development of reflective practice.

The PPDP gives you the strategic direction for education and development whilst the PDPs are formed by combining the needs of the practice with your needs, interest and aspirations as an individual. This workbook provides an opportunity for professional development to become an exciting and dynamic process, which is learner centred, based on wants and needs and gives an opportunity to continuously improve our practice.

What are the best ways to learn?

There are many different styles of learning, some more enjoyable than others. There is no one method or technique that is best. GPs and health professionals are unique professionals and may have developed their own preferred style of learning, which may include reading, reflecting, planning and doing. We tend to learn best when we reflect on our practice (a proforma to help you with this can be found on p. 51). Reflective practice is often at its most powerful when examining significant events (see p. 114). If you are unsure about your own personal learning style, this workbook gives information on how to obtain The Learning Styles Helper's Guide (p. 80) which is designed to increase your insight.

Even when educational needs are met, such positive experiences may not feed back into practice because of various barriers (e.g. time, cost or opportunity). The challenge here is to make CPD work by ensuring that educational events produce demonstrable clinical quality improvement effects. Adopting an ongoing system of monitoring and appraisal will also ensure that progress and development can be measured and assessed, further enhancing personal and professional development.

We should also remember that education can be intrinsically rewarding and fun!

The use of portfolios in learning

A portfolio of learning is a collection of evidence that learning has taken place. It is a physical product of the learning process and gives documentary proof of learning.

To build a portfolio you need to:

1 Identify what you are seeking to learn. (This may change over time and that is fine; changes will need to be documented.)
2 Decide how you can achieve your goals, e.g. by reading, attending lectures, visiting a particular organization or using a new computer program.
3 Document the learning you achieve.
4 Write reflectively and critically about your learning experiences and their outcomes (an audiotape would be an alternative to writing but it must still be both reflective and critical).

In order to achieve steps 3 and 4 you might, for example, put the following into your portfolio:

1 notes of a lecture you attended on the topic you wish to learn about;
2 a tape recording and commentary on a radio programme on teaching or on a medical topic;
3 a list of new ideas you have gained from the above activities to use in your teaching or gained in your work with patients; and
4 an analysis of how well the ideas worked, what helped and hindered the changes you made, how the students or patients reacted to your new approach.

The analysis is a key part of the documentation of your learning as shown below:

> A personal diary or log may be part of your portfolio. Indeed, this is often an exceedingly valuable way of recording and commenting on your thoughts and feelings. If you wish to use your portfolio for accreditation, to offer an interview panel, etc., you may wish to remove these more personal documents. If your portfolio is not going to be seen by anyone else you can, of course, include whatever you choose. In both cases the notes are merely a guide to what may be involved in building a portfolio.

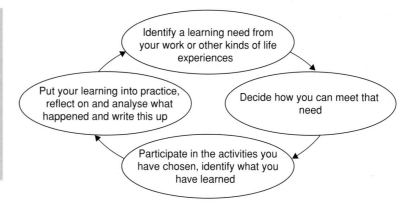

Reflective practice

- How can I convert what I have learned into practice?
- How can patient care be improved as a result of my learning?

These are the central questions of reflective practice. So often, we learn without considering how to apply this learning in practice. We can learn formally, such as in lectures, seminars and from books or protocols, and informally, from colleagues and experiences. However, we learn that we need to take time to consider what it means not only for us, but to the team with whom we work, the wider community, and our patients to continuously improve our practice as shown below:

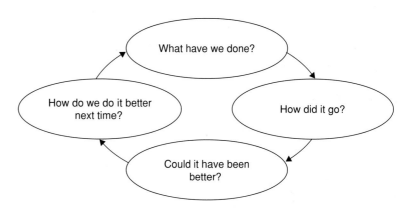

Developing your learning

When you have learned something significant to your clinical practice – be it a skill, some new knowledge, or a change in attitude or approach – you need to take time to think through:

- Were my learning objectives met?
- What have I learned from this event?

The next logical steps could then be:

- What do I want to change as a result of what I have learned?
- What changes, if any, will I make to my practice as a result of my learning?
- What do I need to involve implementing these changes?
- What might stop this happening?
- Can I define the actions needed to bring about change?

A form to help you with this is over the page.

> Let us take an example. You have attended a study session, and learned that the incidence of Chlamydia infection in young people is rising fast. You know that this is a condition that is both preventable and treatable. You have a pang of guilt when you try to recall the last time you discussed this disease, or arranged tests, for a susceptible patient. You know your practice needs to improve.

But how to do this?

At this point you need to sit down for a few minutes and ask yourself the key questions above. In this example, you might decide to discuss your concerns with the PHCT, find out what others do, perhaps by visiting another clinic or practice; seek protocols or guidelines appropriate to your situation; and propose action points to your team. You will need to review progress, and record this in your learning log. Writing down your thoughts and planned actions in a structured way will help ensure they are implemented, especially when you develop the habit of regularly reviewing progress.

Remember, learning does not happen in a vacuum. It is part of your development as a professional, and the ultimate beneficiaries of this process should be your patients.

REFLECTIVE PRACTICE

Event:

Date:

What were my personal learning objectives of this event?

Were my learning objectives met?

What have I learned from this event?

What do I want to change as a result of what I have learned?

What changes, if any, will I make to my practice as a result of my learning?

Who do I need to involve implementing these changes?

What might stop this happening?

Can I define the actions needed to bring about change?

Local delivery plans and health needs assessment
The local delivery plan (LDP)

LDPs are 3-year strategic plans for PCOs and their partners, including local authorities and is both a process for planning and a communication mechanism for informing interested parties.

Each PCO has to produce an LDP for the population area it covers. It will be subject to monitoring of performance and progress against targets stated within the plan, and the effectiveness of partnership working within the health community and with neighbouring health communities.

Organisations such as NHS Trusts that provide services to several PCO areas face significant challenges if PCOs present differing priorities for investment. PCOs themselves need to work collaboratively and develop an approach that ensures consistency in the priorities stated within their individual LDPs where they apply to the commissioning of services from a shared provider. PCOs must balance these collaborative decisions against the needs of their local community and in some circumstances may even have to sacrifice a small local gain for a larger health network gain.

Each PCO will (by their diverse nature) have different organisational arrangements for decision-making and prioritising their work programme.

Practice staff wishing to contribute to the PCO planning process should contact their local PCO for details of how their particular planning framework operates. An absolute essential in planning health services is the participation of clinical professionals at the forefront of the planning process.

The principles of a practice developing a PPDP are the same as a PCO developing its LDP and are a way of expressing your identified health needs priorities.

1 The process should be inclusive; those responsible for delivering the service should have an opportunity to contribute to identifying the issues and developing the solutions, and this gives them ownership. Patients and carers using the service are also able to contribute ideas and observations from their perspective.

2 Any developments should be based on robust information and with regards to meeting the health needs of your patients this will mean undertaking a health need assessment, which is described below. The outcome of your health need assessment can also contribute to the wider PCO picture.

What is a health needs assessment (HNA)?

It is a judgement formed by the understanding of a practice population's benefit in terms of health gain:

- ranging from provision of services through to prevention and palliative care; and
- based on a knowledge of:
  - incidence and prevalence of diseases;
  - effective intervention; and
  - a profile of the population studied.

What are its benefits?

It enables you to identify the needs of your practice population and set and prioritise both the short- and long-term objectives which will be the basis of your PPDP.

It also:
- provides a method of sifting through endless priorities;

- focuses attention on key tasks;
- gives a degree of control and ownership through choosing priorities and targets;
- allows the creation of an action plan to achieve these objectives which will then form the basis for your PPDP; and
- puts team working skills into practice.

What is involved?

1 Creating a profile of your practice population (see p. 54).
2 Identification of key features of your practice population (see p. 56).
3 Identification of top health problems in your practice (see p. 58).
4 Prioritising the list (see p. 62).
5 Planning interventions (see p. 64).
6 Creating an action plan (see p. 68).
7 New priorities (see p. 71).

Your PCO should be able to help you with necessary statistics.

1 CREATING A PROFILE OF YOUR PRACTICE POPULATION

Urban/rural or mixed	Mixed
Demographic features	11% of practice population have chronic illness High proportion of one parent families
Employment/unemployment levels	Low unemployment
Local employers	Westinghouse light industry, agricultural, commuters to Bath, Bristol and London
Access to services (i.e. transport facilities)	One in five has no car, poor public transport Village link operates
What is it like to live here?	Some rural poverty but mostly middle class and affluent, nice countryside but can be isolated. Very good doctors!

The age/sex spread of the practice population

Age groups	0–4	5–16	17–24	25–34	35–44	45–54	55–64	65–74	75–84	85–89	90+
Males	101	266	135	245	338	314	206	181	71	13	6
Females	130	288	118	296	315	308	202	161	110	26	17
Total both sexes	231	554	253	541	653	622	408	342	181	39	23

Figures from age/sex register on 05/06/2005

Population trends

March 2001	3487
March 2002	3553
March 2003	3612
March 2004	3759
March 2005	3850

Is the population increasing or decreasing?

Increasing slowly

What are the reasons?

New housing development

1 CREATING A PROFILE OF YOUR PRACTICE POPULATION

Urban/rural or mixed	
Demographic features	
Employment/unemployment levels	
Local employers	
Access to services (i.e. transport facilities)	
What is it like to live here?	

The age/sex spread of the practice population

Age groups	0–4	5–16	17–24	25–34	35–44	45–54	55–64	65–74	75–84	85–89	90+
Males											
Females											
Total both sexes											

Figures from age/sex register on . . .

Population trends

March 2001		Is the population increasing or decreasing?
March 2002		
March 2003		What are the reasons?
March 2004		
March 2005		

2 KEY FEATURES OF YOUR PRACTICE POPULATION

Causes of substantial mortality

Coronary heart disease

Cancer

Stroke

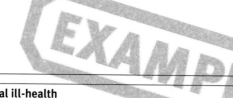

Causes of substantial ill-health

Smoking

Asthma

Ischaemic heart disease

Hypertension

Obesity

Diabetes

Areas of concern

High rates of hospitalisation

Substance dependency

Health needs of 15–24 year olds

Accidents under 5 s

Accidents over 75 s

Dignity and comfort for the terminally ill

Support for carers

Other considerations

NSFs

PCO priorities

LDPs

2 KEY FEATURES OF YOUR PRACTICE POPULATION

Causes of substantial mortality

Causes of substantial ill-health

Areas of concern

Other considerations

3 IDENTIFICATION OF TOP HEALTH PROBLEMS IN YOUR PRACTICE

List the top health problems in your practice. These may include priorities that you can influence directly, or priorities on which you might have to work with others, e.g. voluntary organisations, social services, local schools, etc.

Involve the whole team in completing the questionnaire on the following pages and take account of:

- National priorities – e.g. NSFs
- PCO priorities
- LDPs
- Practice disease and morbidity register
- PHCTs knowledge
- Philosophy of the practice

You may also wish to consider the following topics:
- Smoking cessation
- Drugs and alcohol
- Teenage pregnancy
- Cancer
- Coronary heart disease/stroke
- Diabetes
- Respiratory health
- Waiting lists and times
- Access to GP/primary health care professional
- Mental health
- Older people's services
- Children's services
- Patient and carer involvement
- Occupational health and safety
- Premises
- Disability Discrimination Act (1995) compliance
- IM&T including Caldicott
- Practice professional development and training plan

---

1 Description of the practice population

High elderly population

Rural occupations – farming community

Low unemployment

Predominantly middle class

Limited public transport/poor access to services

Commuters

Drug and alcohol abuse

EXAMPLE

---

2 Based on our own experience, are there key things that stick out as health problems in our practice?

Elderly isolated

Commuters – work in London, live in Wiltshire (unable to attend surgery appointments)

Diabetes

Asthma admissions

Coronary heart disease

Prevalence of depression seems low – Are we missing something?

Dependence on health services

3 How do you think these differ from other areas/practices?

Predominantly middle class – health care dependency

Rural/isolated areas

Higher elderly population

4 What things help people feel healthy here?

Fresh air/pleasant, friendly environment/rural, picturesque countryside

Caring services

Good housing

Supportive neighbours

Access to sport centres and gyms

Exercise

5 What stops people feeling healthy?

Isolation

Access to surgery

Access to services (e.g. social services, NHS)

Access to shops

Motorways

Pylons

Drug and alcohol dependency

6 Are there key things that could be done to improve people's health?

Improve public transport

Advice about accident prevention and health
lifestyles

Access to link worker

More effective use of health visitor

Access to surgery

Drug and alcohol abuse counsellor

7 Are there key things the practice could do to improve people's health?

Improve care of chronic disease, diabetes, chronic
obstructive pulmonary disease

Opportunistic advice about lifestyles

Opportunistic screening regarding family histories

Extend surgery hours to provide appointments for
commuters

More nurse-led chronic disease management clinics

Publicise self-help groups

Drug and alcohol dependency clinics

3 IDENTIFICATION OF TOP HEALTH PROBLEMS IN YOUR PRACTICE

1 Description of the practice population

2 Based on our own experience, are there key things that stick out as health problems in our practice?

3 How do you think these differ from other areas/practices?

4 What things help people feel healthy here?

5 What stops people feeling healthy?

6 Are there key things that could be done to improve people's health?

7 Are there key things the practice could do to improve people's health?

4 PRIORITISING THE LIST

Involve all PHCT members, and remember those who are attached to your practice and/or part-time members of the PHCT.

Apply your chosen criteria to select three or four areas on which to focus attention in the coming year.

Ask the following questions of each health need identified	CAN WE IMPROVE THE FOLLOWING HEALTH NEEDS?		
	Prevention of coronary heart disease?	Care of patients with asthma?	Care for housebound diabetic patients?
Interest to whole team	4	3	3
Achievable with available resources	3	4	4
Easily identified group	4	3	4
Recognisable benefits to the whole team	4	4	4
Effectiveness of interventions, e.g. health outcomes	4	4	2
Worth doing something about – prevalence	4	4	4
How much energy is needed	4	4	3
Importance to Community	4	4	4
Total	31	29	28

As a result of this exercise what are we going to choose to go on to our PPDP?

Secondary prevention of coronary heart disease

Key	
0	Does not meet criteria
1	
2	
3	
4	Meets criteria

4 PRIORITISING THE LIST

	CAN WE IMPROVE THE FOLLOWING HEALTH NEEDS?		
Ask the following questions of each health need identified			
Interest to whole team			
Achievable with available resources			
Easily identified group			
Recognisable benefits to the whole team			
Effectiveness of interventions, e.g. health outcomes			
Worth doing something about – prevalence			
How much energy is needed			
Importance to Community			
Total			

As a result of this exercise what are we going to choose to go on to our PPDP?

Key

0	Does not meet criteria
1	
2	
3	
4	Meets criteria

5 PLANNING INTERVENTIONS

HEALTH PROBLEM: SECONDARY PREVENTION OF CORONARY HEART DISEASE

CHECKING OUT ASSUMPTIONS

What information do we have on this health problem?

Diagnoses; risk factors; admissions; operations

How accessible is the information, e.g. paper notes, on computer?

QOF and the need to demonstrate clinical care, this is probably available on computer

What information might we need to collect in the future?

Items in NSF not covered by QOF

COLLECTING INFORMATION

How easy is it to extract information, e.g. prescribing referrals, risk factors?

QMAS will collect QOF data. PACT will provide additional material. PCO and/or acute trust may provide info on referrals and admissions

Do we wish to set up systems to collect other necessary information?

If we deem the information is 'necessary' then it can be added to existing templates

What services are currently provided for this health problem?

Practice clinics; support groups; practice-linked exercise groups

If services are currently provided who provides them?

Practice nurses; specialist nurses at acute trusts; local gyms in cooperation with practices and/or PCOs

What are appropriate interventions for this problem?

Advice, investigations, drug treatment and referral

What might we provide in the practice differently to meet this health need?

Education sessions for patient groups – in the evenings to allow those who still work to attend

What other resources can we tap into?

Online leaflets for patients; data analysis by PRIMIS

How will we know that things have improved?

By setting up an audit cycle – where are we now; where do we want to be and when; what changes do we need to make; implement; measure again

5 PLANNING INTERVENTIONS

HEALTH PROBLEM: SECONDARY PREVENTION OF CORONARY HEART DISEASE

CHECKING OUT ASSUMPTIONS:

What information do we have on this health problem?

How accessible is the information, e.g. paper notes, on computer?

What information might we need to collect in the future?

COLLECTING INFORMATION

How easy is it to extract information, e.g. prescribing referrals, risk factors?

Do we wish to set up systems to collect other necessary information?

What services are currently provided for this health problem?

If services are currently provided who provides them?

What are appropriate interventions for this problem?

What might we provide in the practice differently to meet this health need?

What other resources can we tap into?

How will we know that things have improved?

6 CREATING AN ACTION PLAN

Having established the needs of your practice population, you will need to develop the action plans that will form your PPDP.

Action plans do not need to be documents with huge amounts of narrative. It is important that the PHCT focus on what they want to achieve and how they are to implement the change.

Action plans should include:

Objectives

What is the main objective? What links does the objective have to other plans and strategies?

Current position

How the service is currently provided, current activity, cost and what are the issues?

Responsibilities

Who will be involved/responsible for implementing the actions? (*This must be explicit!*)

Actions

How will they meet the objective?

Timetable

Target dates for achievement of the actions

Resource implications

What is required in terms of resources (staff, equipment, facilities, time, training etc.) in order for the objectives to be achievable?

Evaluation

What was successful?

What was not so successful and why?

What might be done differently in future?

Objective: Secondary Prevention of Coronary Heart Disease

Who will be involved?:
Clinical staff supported by administrative staff **Lead:**

How will this be done?
• Ensure accuracy of disease register currently held on EMIS version 4 • Baseline assessment to see where we are now • Establish evidence-based computer template for secondary prevention of chronic heart disease • Generate recall letters, advising patients that the practice would like to review them every 6 months • Record attendance with results of investigations and examination findings on computer template • Audit of non-attenders every 3 months with reminder letters sent • Annual audit of clinical effectiveness against key markers, e.g. diastolic blood pressure, smoking, cholesterol, BMI, exercise, aspirin, etc.

By When?
Priority Year 1

What was successful?
Disease register for coronary heart disease sorted out 98% of target group had blood pressure checked and smoking status recorded Cholesterol fallen over the year and all patients without contraindications were on aspirin

What was not so successful and why?
Percentage of smokers still the same (smoke stop clinic on Monday morning)

What might we do differently in future?
Rationalise our statin prescribing Arrange a more convenient smoke stop clinic

6 CREATING AN ACTION PLAN

Objective:

Who will be involved?:

Lead:

How will this be done?

By when?

What was successful?

What was not so successful and why?

What might we do differently in future?

7 NEW PRIORITIES

Once we have tackled secondary prevention of coronary heart disease, we plan to do the same for asthma and diabetic patients.

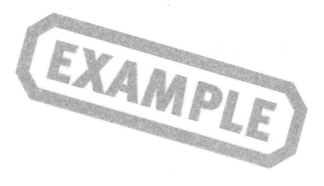

You can continually build on the LDPs and your practice's HNA by evaluating whether you should continue with the same priorities on a longer term basis, or set new priorities for the following year. This should be completed in conjunction with your PPDP and be part of your annual planning cycle.

7 NEW PRIORITIES

You can continually build on the LDPs and your practice's HNA by evaluating whether you should continue with the same priorities on a longer term basis, or set new priorities for the following year. This should be completed in conjunction with your PPDP and be part of your annual planning cycle.

Developing the primary health care team

Primary health care teams (PHCTs)

The concept of the PHCT has been in existence for almost 50 years. The drive has been to encourage closer working between these staff and the staff of general practice, regardless of their varying employers, and different reports through that time have examined ways of making the team work more efficiently and effectively. Whether the team can be successful has depended upon the physical geography of the bases/buildings, but time after time one of the main barriers to efficient working has been the fact that staff have had different employers: the Health Authority (now the PCO) general practice and social services. Without doubt the most successful PHCTs have been those where all barriers have been dropped and all staff treat each other with mutual professional respect.

For a busy GP or practice nurse valuable time can be saved and a better patient service offered where each patient contact is maximised; however in reality, time and other conflicts can and do occur. To be truly effective your practice/business manager should also be part of the PHCT and they can best advise how to overcome any such obstacles. In most cases, the presence of a single GP and practice nurse to represent their discipline's views within the PHCT is quite sufficient. Some PCOs make specific funding available for PHCT involvement – your practice/business manager will be able to advise you on this.

Some PHCTs have a permanent funded clinical lead and/or a rotating chairperson to call, run, record and distribute recommendations from meetings.

How to get the most from the PHCT?

Whilst to some extent this will depend on the existing contractual relationships, consider this:

> Time invested = better relationships and better results.

For your practice and your patients to gain the most from the PHCT, there need to be a set of agreed criteria both in terms of the PHCTs clinical focus and the time that members will commit to the PHCT; remember, it is unlikely that only GPs will be under time pressures. Ask other team members for their input and how they feel about the team whilst remembering to praise past achievements and recognise commitment; you may be able to achieve this at one well-chaired meeting if a detailed agenda is prepared and sent out in sufficient time for team members to be able to prepare for the meeting. If this is not possible, you may need to consider the need for a PHCT away day or half day to agree the way ahead but these meetings are costly in terms of missed appointments and the need for such a commitment must be agreed with a majority of team members before making such a commitment. One factor that will affect the amount of time needed will be the size of the PHCT as everyone present must feel involved and there must be sufficient time for them to contribute, comment and reflect.

What are away days?

Away days or half-day get-togethers for entire practices, although still a relatively new idea, are on the increase. Depending on the size and geography of your PHCT, plan well ahead to ensure adequate clinical coverage. Patients need to be kept informed of both the closure and the reasons for it. Do not forget to include all staff and other professionals attached and associated to the practice in the away day process. If they and other staff are unable to attend, then a feedback session after the event would be helpful.

Why have away days?

Away days can be used to bring together various pieces of work in order to agree as a team on the priorities for the coming year.

What can be achieved?

- Identification of clinical and organizational priorities.
- Identification of skills to meet these priorities.
- Identification of gaps and overlaps in service provision.
- Recommendations for addressing the gaps and overlaps in provision.

An example of a practice away day programme, ground rules and helpful information on running small groups follows.

AWAY DAY PROGRAMME

9.30 a.m.
Welcome and expectations of the day
Theme:
Where are we now?
Where do we want to be?
How are we going to get there?

Ground rules (p. 76)
Ice breaker: Learning styles (p. 80)

10.30 a.m.
Where are we now?
Practice SCOT analysis (p. 79)
What has gone well?
What could we do better?
What could we improve upon?

12.15 p.m. Lunch

'Vision of the Future'

1 p.m.
Where do we want to be?
Pairs/group brainstorm
What gets in the way?
What are the solutions?

3 p.m.
How are we going to get there?
• Discuss, agree and prioritise the PPDP
• Identification of key action areas for individuals or team
• Action plan – who does what? By when?
• Date of review

4.30 p.m.
Reflection on the day and close

Ground rules for away days

- Listen to each other, do not interrupt, give opportunities for all to contribute, show you are listening and respect the other members of the group.
- Confidentiality.
- Personal honesty.
- Be honest in a constructive way.
- Be open.
- Keep to the point.
- Keep it simple/no jargon.
- Make your own statements.
- Do not be too ambitious.
- Finish on time.

What do you want from today?

The following pointers might be helpful:

- clarity about the way forward as a PHCT;
- strengthen the PHCT;
- provide a shared understanding of the PHCT;
- establish where we are starting from;
- feel more part of the team;
- feel that as a team we are aiming at same goals (know what the goals are);
- share the barriers;
- form a vision/practice plan;
- allow the opportunity to develop a shared vision – practice development and individual needs – produce something tangible;
- time to develop personally; and
- individual development needs/skills.

Running small groups

In this type of activity the group relies principally on its own members as resources and will meet several times to cover a topic in various sections. Take, for example, *palliative care* or *chronic disease management*. There would be an aim, say, '*to improve the care of patients with chronic disease*'. This would best be broken down into objectives.

- To increase the number of post-MI patients taking aspirin.
- To increase the number of post-MI patients taking a statin.
- To ensure all patients with chronic obstructive pulmonary disease have had a spirometry maximal peak expiratory flow recorded annually.
- To ensure all patients with diabetes have annual retinal screening.

> '**SMART**' can be a useful mnemonic:
> Specific, Measurable, Agreed, Realistic and Time-based.

 Remember that an aim is a general expression of intent and an objective is measurable and subsequently open to audit.

Small groups can be exceptionally inventive, effective, cohesive and collaborative. Equally, they can be uncomfortable, acrimonious and emotionally fraught. Good leadership will enhance the possibilities for success and reduce the risk of disaster. Most people, but not all, can work effectively in small groups.

Tips on running small groups

- The group should have constant membership of between 5 and 13, the ideal being about 8.
- Ensure all group members know each other or introduce themselves.
- All members to have equal rank (no doctors and nurses, just people with special skills, knowledge or attitude).
- The task should be agreed and clarified.
- Do not have two conversations at one time.
- Allow everyone to speak without interruption.
- Encourage the noisy to 'tone down'.
- Encourage the quiet to 'switch on'; they are used to being ignored, let them feel their opinion is as important as anyone else's.
- Encourage honesty.
- Gently discourage boastfulness.
- No 'telling tales out of school'; whatever is said in a group must be confidential.
- Provide emotional support when appropriate.
- Give intellectual challenges when appropriate.
- Value openly each member's contribution.

Brainstorming

Purpose

- To increase creative skills.
- To provide a useful technique for team problem-solving.

  This activity helps to clarify personal goals, improve problem-solving skills, increase creativity and develop team-building skills.

Method

The technique of brainstorming can be applied in many ways. The activity can be modified to suit different needs because it is the basic method that is important. To obtain the best results, it is important to follow the rules as closely as possible.

1 Set aside at least half an hour for the activity.
2 Decide on a subject in which change and/or creativity are important. This should be a topic of interest or importance to the group. The topic should be stated as a problem, question or objective.
3 Explain that 'brainstorming' is a process in which all members of the group are invited to suggest as many ideas as they can. Make it clear that *all* ideas, no matter how absurd they may appear, will be recorded and that there will be no evaluation of the ideas during the first stage; as soon as an idea is introduced, it will be recorded, and the next idea will be introduced.
4 When everyone understands the guidelines, allow some time for the participants to ask questions. Then begin the brainstorming session by writing the chosen topic clearly on the flip chart, e.g. How can we improve communication between members of the PHCT?
5 Have the members brainstorm the topic for at least 5 minutes and list (without any discussion) *every* idea suggested. Two or three flip charts may be used to record ideas, which are likely to come thick and fast when there is a rule prohibiting evaluation or censorship.

6   Divide the participants into two groups and ask each group to decide which suggestion falls into each of two categories: *'Very Relevant'* and *'Potentially Relevant'*. Allow up to half an hour for this task.

7   Ask each group to list all the *'Very Relevant'* ideas on one sheet and all the *'Potentially Relevant'* ideas on a second sheet.

8   Have the groups meet together and share their lists. Ask individuals to examine the lists and to choose the suggestions that could make the greatest contribution to solving the problem or achieving the objective.

9   Take the suggestions with the highest scores and produce a written plan to implement them (the example given below may help).

10 After a suitable period of time, during which implementation is tried, have the group meet again to discuss how well the plans are progressing and to take any necessary corrective action.

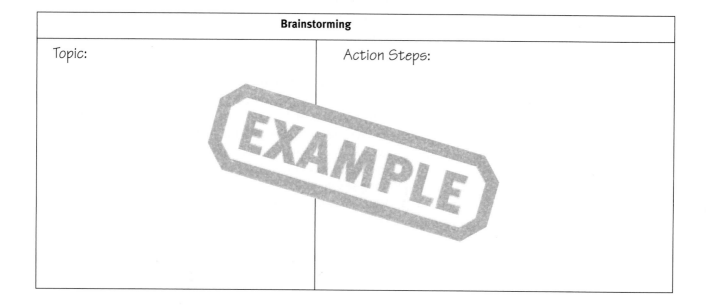

Brainstorming	
Topic: How can we improve communication between members of the PHCT?	**Action Steps:** PHCT meeting every month in protected time One alternative Wednesday and Friday afternoons employ locum to cover GMS. Each and every patient contact to be recorded on the computer: • Surgery appointments • Home visits • Telephone calls • Any discussion between members of the PHCT • Copy internal e-mail to keep everyone informed

Brainstorming	
Topic:	Action Steps:

Practice SCOT analysis

Strengths and challenges are things that exist for you and your practice at this moment. Opportunities and threats are possibilities that may come along in the future, but that need to be thought about now. You will need to maximise your strengths and opportunities and minimise your challenges and threats.

Developing a SCOT analysis could involve individual or all members of the practice team.

- **Strengths** relate to achievements over the year.
- **Challenges** highlight any difficulties or obstacles that have been experienced.
- **Opportunities** lists factors that will influence the success of individuals, team and practice, i.e. ideas for the future.
- **Threats** lists things that may be an obstacle to development.

An example could be:

Strengths	Challenges
• Stable patient population • Hard-working and effective PHCT • Dispensing • Paperless practice	• Demanding patients • Elderly list • Appointments with multiple problems • Prevalence of chronic disease • Rural isolation • Keeping up with changing goal posts • Skills mix of PHCT
Opportunities	**Threats**
• PMS pilot • Dispensing • Maximising QOF points • Developing nurses to take on further roles, triage, etc. • Partners work outside practice, e.g. sports medicine, police, clinical assistant	• Insufficient appointment time • Increase in list size • Workload • Burnout

Developing learning profiles for PHCTs

This will:
- enable the team to learn together for the benefit of patients and themselves;
- develop consistent standards for patient care;
- build professional confidence; and
- enable team members to articulate their achievements.

What can you do for your team?

- Actively seek opportunities to learn together, i.e. have regular clinical meetings, encourage *Significant-event auditing* (see p. 114) and promote multidisciplinary review of clinical practice.
- Encourage everyone to discover their own learning style. Information on how to obtain Honey and Mumford's *The Learning Styles Helper's Guide* and *The Learning Styles Questionnaire 80 item version* can be found below.
- Encourage everyone to reflect on their particular learning style. Encourage the PHCT to complete the *Reflecting on Learning Styles* pro forma on page 82.

The Learning Styles Helper's Guide

Given the same experience, why do some people learn while others do not? A major reason is that people differ in the way they prefer to learn.

The Learning Styles Helper's Guide (Honey & Mumford 2000) includes:
- Description of the learning cycle and the four styles: activist, reflector, theorist and pragmatist; for further information on the four styles see below.
- A variety of norms against which results can be compared.
- Suggestions on how trainers can use the information to:
  - design events to cover the complete learning cycle;
  - select activities to suit different preferences; and
  - help individuals to strengthen underutilised styles.
- Suggestions on how people can better manage their learning.
  Each guide costs £16.95.

  The Learning Styles Questionnaire 80 item version includes the questionnaire and score key, and all the supporting information for the individual learner. The cost of each booklet depends on the number purchased but start with a minimum order of 10 at £6.50 each.

  For further information on *The Learning Styles Helper's Guide* and *The Learning Styles Questionnaire 80 item version*, Personal Workbooks and Learning Logs, contact Peter Honey Publications, Ardingly House, 10 Linden Avenue, Maidenhead, Berks, SL6 6HB (Tel 01628 633946; Fax 01628 633262; e-mail info@peterhoney.co.uk).

Honey and Mumford identified four learning styles as follows

Activists

Activists involve themselves fully and without bias in new experiences. They enjoy the 'here and now' and are happy to be dominated by immediate experiences. They are open-minded and not sceptical, which tends to make them enthusiastic about anything new. Their philosophy is: 'I'll try anything once'. They tend to act first and consider the consequences afterwards. Their days are filled with activity. They tackle problems by brainstorming. As soon as the excitement from one activity has died down, they are busy looking for the next. They tend to thrive on the challenge of new experiences but are bored with implementation and longer term consolidation. They are gregarious people constantly involving themselves with others, but in doing so they seek to centre all activities on themselves.

Reflectors

Reflectors like to stand back to ponder experiences and observe from many different perspectives. They collect data, both first-hand and from others, and prefer to think about it thoroughly before coming to any conclusion. The thorough collection and analysis of data about experiences and events are what counts, so they tend to postpone reaching definitive conclusions for as long as possible. Their philosophy is to be cautious. They are thoughtful people who like to consider all possible angles and implications before making a move and prefer to take a back seat in meetings and discussions. They enjoy observing other people in action. They listen to others and get the drift of the discussion before making their own points. They tend to adopt a low profile and have a slightly distant, tolerant, unruffled air about them. When they act it is part of a wide picture which includes the past, the present and others' observations as well as their own.

Theorists

Theorists adapt and integrate observations into complex but logically sound theories. They think problems through in a vertical, step-by-step logical way. They assimilate disparate facts into coherent theories. They tend to be perfectionists who will not rest easy until things are tidy and fit into a rational scheme. They like to analyse and synthesise. They are keen on basic assumptions, principles, theories, models and systems thinking. Their philosophy prizes rationality and logic. 'If it's logical it's good.' Questions they frequently ask are: 'Does it make sense?' 'How does this fit with that?' 'What are the basic assumptions?' They tend to be detached, analytical and dedicated to rational objectivity rather than anything subjective or ambiguous. Their approach to problems is consistently logical. This is their 'mental set' and they rigidly reject anything that does not fit within it. They prefer to maximise certainty and feel uncomfortable with subjective judgements, lateral thinking and anything flippant.

Pragmatists

Pragmatists are keen on trying out ideas, theories and techniques to see if they work in practice. They positively search out new ideas and take the first opportunity to experiment with applications. They are the sort of people who return from management courses brimming with new ideas that they want to try out in practice. They like to get on with things and act quickly and confidently on ideas that attract them. They tend to be impatient with ruminating and open-ended discussions. They are essentially practical, down-to-earth people who like making practical decisions and solving problems. They respond to problems and opportunities 'as a challenge'. Their philosophy is 'There is always a better way' and 'If it works it's good'.

REFLECTING ON LEARNING STYLE QUESTIONNAIRE

Now reflect on your particular learning style. Are you an activist, reflector, theorist or pragmatist?

Give an example of how your learning style may influence an aspect of decision-making in your practice

Using knowledge of this learning style what may be the best way to present an educational event that would maximise your learning and enjoyment?

Do you consider this to be true of your practice in general?

What does this preferred learning style suggest about the way you respond to changes in general practice?

Can you give a recent example of this?

How do you describe the preferred learning style of your practice?

Does this differ from your individual learning style?

If so, how might a compromise be reached in terms of an effective provision of an educational event for your practice?

Skill mix of the primary health care team

What is skill mix?

Skill mix is 'identifying the range of tasks and responsibilities involved in providing care within a particular speciality, what levels are involved and therefore who is appropriate to carry them out'. The World Health Organisation has defined it as 'usually used to describe the mix of posts or occupations in an organisation. It may also refer to the combinations of activities or skills needed for each job within the organisation' (Zurn *et al.* 2002).

The skill mix review of your current team can help once you have identified the team's priorities.

Ask each member of the team to measure their skills on the standards for assessment competence scale 'novice to expert' (Benner 1984).

Level 1	'Novice' No knowledge or working experience
Level 2	'Advanced beginner' Some knowledge and limited working experience. Needs help in setting priorities Can demonstrate marginally acceptable performance
Level 3	'Competent' Conscious deliberate planning is characteristic of this skill level Becoming skilled but lacks the speed and flexibility to be totally proficient
Level 4	'Proficient' Has an experience-based ability to recognise whole situations and therefore knows when the expected normal does not occur and modifies responses accordingly
Level 5	'Expert' Enormous background knowledge and significant level of skill Focus on the nature of the problem without wasting time on unfruitful alternative diagnoses and solutions May use analytical tools when the need to generate alternative perspectives (creativity) is needed

INDIVIDUAL SKILLS ASSESSMENT (CLINICAL)

Name:

Dr P Spooner

Post:

GP Partner

Core skills	Level 1	Level 2	Level 3	Level 4	Level 5
Consultation skills					✓
Diagnosis					✓
Treatment					✓
Special interests					
Paediatrics				✓	
Cardiology			✓		
Gastroenterology				✓	
Specialist skills					
Child health surveillance					✓
Echogardiograms				✓	
Gastroscopy					✓
Flexible sigmoidoscopy				✓	

INDIVIDUAL SKILLS ASSESSMENT (CLINICAL)

Name:

Post:

Core skills	Level 1	Level 2	Level 3	Level 4	Level 5
Special interests					
Specialist skills					

INDIVIDUAL SKILLS ASSESSMENT
(NON-CLINICAL TEAM MEMBERS)

Name:

John Brown

Post:

Business/Practice Manager

Core skills	Level 1	Level 2	Level 3	Level 4	Level 5
Financial plan					✓
Business management					✓
HSAW/COSHH				✓	
Special interests					
Significant event audit					✓
Contingency planning					✓
Specialist skills					
Staff selection					✓
IT					✓
Employment/European law					✓

INDIVIDUAL SKILLS ASSESSMENT
(NON-CLINICAL TEAM MEMBERS)

Name:

Post:

Core skills	Level 1	Level 2	Level 3	Level 4	Level 5
Special interests					
Specialist skills					

TEAM SKILLS ASSESSMENT

Name	Core skills and special interests	Specialist skills	Level of specialist skills				
			1	2	3	4	5
GP1	Generic general practice	Asthma					✓
	Paediatrics	Child health surveillance					✓
	General medicine	Diabetes			✓		
		Cardiology				✓	
		Epilepsy			✓		
GP2	Generic general practice						✓
	O&G	Ultrasound				✓	
		Sexual disease screening				✓	
		Colposcopy				✓	
	Gastroenterology	Sigmoidoscopy					✓
GP3	Generic general practice						✓
	Surgery	Minor surgery				✓	
	Psychiatry	Section 12 approved				✓	
		Counselling				✓	
Practice nurse	Generic nursing skills	Travel vaccinations					✓
		Family planning				✓	
	Chronic disease management	Diabetes				✓	
		Hypertension				✓	
		Asthma			✓		
Community nurse 1	Generic community nursing skills	Wound management					✓

Name	Core skills and special interests	Specialist skills	Level of specialist skills				
			1	2	3	4	5
		Treatment of leg ulcers				✓	
		Infection control				✓	
	ITU bank nurse	High-dependency patients			✓		
Community nurse 2	Generic community nursing skills						✓
	McMillan trained	Palliative care					✓
	Ex-urology ward sister	Continence advice				✓	
Health visitor	Generic nursing and health visitor skills	Child development				✓	
		Accident prevention			✓		
		Health education					✓
	MSc in education	Teaching					✓
		Nurse mentor				✓	
Business/ Practice Manager 1	Financial planning	Budget forecasting					✓
		Cost-effectiveness of change			✓		
		Accounts, payrolls and NHS pensions					✓
	MBA	Practice manager mentor					✓
		Team working				✓	
Business/ Practice Manager 2	Accountancy	Accounts, payrolls and NHS pensions					✓
		Budgets and cash flow analysis			✓		
		Risk assessment					✓
	MBA	COSHH					✓
		SEA				✓	

TEAM SKILLS ASSESSMENT

Name	Core skills and special interests	Specialist skills	Level of specialist skills				
			1	2	3	4	5

Name	Core skills and special interests	Specialist skills	Level of specialist skills				
			1	2	3	4	5

The next logical steps should be to:
- Identify and define the work that needs to be done to provide the service.
- Determine what responsibilities must be adopted and what tasks done to perform this work well and economically and to achieve specific outcomes.
- Define what mix of general skills and specific skills are required to perform to that level.

?
- Do the skills required fit with the needs of the patients?
- Are there any skills gaps?
- Who in the team has the potential to fill them?
- Would you like to add this to your PPDP or individual PDPs?

Useful websites for *Skill mix of the primary health care team*

Honey and Mumford Learning Styles	www.peterhoney.com/product/ brochure
OECD Paper 'Skill Mix and Policy Change in the Workforce'	www.oecd.org/dataoecd/30/28/ 33857785.pdf
Teamwork and Skill Mix	www.nelh.nhs.uk/nsf/ inprimarycare/organisational _devt/ teamwork.htm

A full list of websites can be found on pages 192–197.

Appraisal

GP NHS appraisal

GP appraisal has been recently introduced across the UK and appears to have been well received by most GPs despite many initial concerns about both the process and content of appraisal.

The current aim is to maintain and improve the quality of appraisal as a supportive developmental tool for professional development, as well as linking it to revalidation in a way that effectively identifies and addresses underperformance. GPs have been engaging in some form of remunerated professional development since the implementation of the GP contract in 1990. However, this was often an opportunistic *ad hoc* process that did not always address the individuals key development needs in a structured way. Appraisal and revalidation provide the opportunity to guide and assess every GP's ongoing professional development, based on learning needs identified through regular reflection and patient and colleague feedback. Delivering two linked processes that identify unacceptable performance in the small minority, whilst developing and maintaining high-quality practice for the majority of GPs, is a key challenge of the next decade of general practice professional development.

Since the first edition of this book in 2000, appraisal has been established as an annual requirement for all GPs. Appraisal was originally developed in the commercial setting as a mechanism for regular performance review, often linked to pay awards. General practice professional partnerships operate differently from hierarchical managed organisations, and this has led to the development of a specific model of appraisal for GPs.

One of these models is based on the School of Health and Related Research (ScHARR) report at Sheffield University, which defined appraisal within general practice as being less about performance and more about:

> exploring role expectations . . . reviewing progress . . . [and] identifying personal development needs. (Martin 2001)
>
> Appraisal was introduced by the Department of Health as a 'formative and developmental process . . . a positive process, to give GPs feedback on their past performance, to chart continuing progress and identify development needs.' (Department of Health 1999)

There has as yet been no full evaluation of the outcomes of appraisal, but there is substantial anecdotal evidence from small-scale PCO surveys, that in general the process has been well received as both useful and supportive. Preliminary reports following the first year of GP appraisals suggest that this aim has often been achieved with comments such as *'This was the first time in my professional career anyone had asked me to reflect on my work or given me feedback on my performance'* appearing on official websites. The challenge now is to build on this positive start and to maintain appraisal as a supportive, formative developmental process, whilst acknowledging that it must also feed into the revalidation process. The report from the Shipman Inquiry (2005) has further reinforced this message.

It is likely that all GPs will be required to produce robust and personally attributable evidence to support their revalidation, in order to assure their employers and the public that they are both fit to practice and up to date in their skills and knowledge.

Preparing for your appraisal

It is highly recommended that all appraisal documentation is completed electronically. This reduces the workload on a year-by-year basis as some of the documentation needs only to be updated not rewritten.

The appraisal forms can be downloaded directly from the DoH website. All the appraisal forms can also be filled in and stored online when you register with the DoH appraisal website.

There are three forms to be completed/updated before each appraisal meeting.

Form 1   Basic appraisee details
Form 2   Current medical activities
Form 3   Material for appraisal

In addition to the above, there are a further two forms to complete following the appraisal:

Form 4   Summary of appraisal discussion with agreed action and personal development plan
Forms 5   (optional) Detailed confidential account of appraisal interview

All of the above forms are available from the GP appraisal website: www.dh.gov.uk/gpappraisal.

Appraisal is based on the GMC's document *Good Medical Practice* (General Medical Council 2001), which describes the principles of good medical practice, and standards of competence, care and conduct expected of doctors in all aspects of their professional work. These are:

- Good clinical care
- Maintaining good medical practice
- Teaching and training
- Relationships with patients
- Working with colleagues
- Probity
- Health

A free CD-ROM video guide to GP appraisal is also available from the NHS response line, quoting reference 28027:

08701 555455

The RCGP has produced an expanded version specifically aimed at GPs and this is obtainable on their website.

Work is currently in progress to define more clearly the 'evidence set' that should support the statements you make in your appraisal forms (Form 3), including the following:

1   Participation in audit and significant event analysis.
2   Retraining in basic cardiopulmonary resuscitation.
3   Regular clinical learning activities.
4   Participation in patient surveys with feedback about the individual GP.
5   Participation in some communication skills training.
6   Description of, and reflection on, any complaints received.

7   An audit of records.

8   Feedback on teaching, research and management activity if appropriate.

9   Some form of 360 degrees feedback from colleagues is likely to become a requirement once existing tools have been validated in the GP context.

Hints

*   Collecting this information during the year rather than just before the appraisal meeting will make the whole process much less stressful. The DoH appraisal website provides templates for recording evidence in each of the sections of Form 3, and it now also allows you to scan in and store relevant papers such as attendance certificates, course records or patient survey reports to provide a complete electronic copy of your appraisal documentation.

*   Prepare for the appraisal interview by identifying the key areas from Form 3 that you feel would be valuable to discuss with your appraiser. This may include things that have been very successful as well as issues that concern or challenge you. Your reflections on what you have achieved and what you have not addressed from last year's PDP are also important areas to be covered in the appraisal discussion.

The appraisal interview

This should be led at least initially by you as the appraisee. It is protected time for you to explore any issues about your professional practice, and for the appraiser to raise any questions they have identified from your appraisal forms and evidence. The appraisal process should conform to agreed local standards – an example of these has been produced by the National Association of Primary Care Educators. You should have adequate notice of the date of your appraisal, with a choice of appraiser and venue. The PCO's policy on confidentiality – the storage and use of anonymised data from Form 4 – should be made clear to you. It may be useful to make note of any key points that emerge during the appraisal interview you feel should be included in the appraisal summary document. Form 4 is completed by your appraiser, but the main action points should be agreed between you and your appraiser at the end of the interview.

After the appraisal interview

Your first task is to correct, amend and countersign Form 4 as an accurate representation of the appraisal discussion. It is worth taking a little time over this and making sure all the important issues have been included as the action points in Form 4 will form the basis for your PDP.

Well-defined educational needs also help your PCO plan educational provision at a district level. Try to make your PDP aims

SMART, i.e. Specific, Measurable, Agreed, Realistic and Time based

'*To attend two outpatient dermatology clinics and prepare an update on current skin disease management by November 2005*' is very much useful and easier to assess in terms of achievement the following year than '*to improve skills in dermatology*'.

A number of practices have also used the outcomes of individual appraisals as a basis for producing a practice development plan. This allows individuals who may have identified similar learning needs in isolation, to plan how these might be jointly met, or to emphasise these in assessing the practice's overall clinical priorities. The GPs also have the opportunity to link each individual's identified learning needs to practice priorities, providing a coherent basis for decisions about funding for courses, time out for additional training, etc. Your PDP is ideally a flexible document that can be added to during the year if new issues arise. Saving it as a desktop icon on your computer makes it easy to be accessed and updated.

The BMJ has set up an excellent website to facilitate GP's learning and professional development. Once registered, you will receive a weekly electronic update of new learning programmes on the site, each of which is designed to be completed in 15–30 minutes, and which can be added to your plan for use at a later date. These activities are stored in your plan and can be printed out each year for your appraisal evidence folder. Many other websites provide electronic learning programmes or signpost you to educational activities in your area – a selection of these are given at the end of this chapter.

Appraisal is an annual review of reflection, learning and review that should form part of every GP's ongoing professional development. Ideally, it is useful to arrange some ongoing contact with your appraiser at some point during the year – this might just be a telephone call or an e-mail to review progress. This will not be possible for all GPs; appraisers change from year to year and many may not have the time to keep any ongoing contact with their appraisees. Setting PDP aims within specific time frames can also be helpful, and some practices have set up informal mentoring arrangements between GP pairs as an incentive for each to demonstrate that their development needs are being addressed.

Appraisal and revalidation

The government has decided to review the GMC's proposed new system of revalidation in the light of Dame Janet Smith's 5th report on the Shipman case. The review includes the role of NHS appraisal and considers the GMC's arrangements for examining a doctor's fitness to practise within the revalidation process. This has also meant that the intended launch of GP revalidation, originally scheduled for April 2005, has been postponed.

However, the following is known even though the review is pending:

Revalidation is being introduced for all UK doctors. It is a five-yearly assessment of whether an individual doctor remains both up to date and fit to practise. Appraisal is not in itself an instrument designed to review performance in a summative way, but 'satisfactory' participation in annual appraisal will be a central component in your recommendation to be revalidated. As the appraisal process evolves it is likely that appraisers will be asked to highlight any early indicators of underperformance to their appraisees, and to guide them towards sources of support that should help to improve performance. Examples of early indicators of underperformance might include consistent failure to address key learning needs identified in your PDP, lack of IT skills in your GP computer system and in accessing web-based learning, very high stress levels due to workload or other pressures. Appraisal should provide the opportunity to feed back on good performance and to support you in any areas that might threaten your licence to practice when you are revalidated. If your appraiser does identify any areas of potential concern then these must be addressed as early as possible, so that progress and change can be monitored at your next appraisal.

Accumulating evidence and taking a little time out on a regular basis to review any new learning needs will make an important contribution to satisfactory participation in appraisal. You will also need to work within your practice or perhaps in a group with other non-practice-based performers to set up a system for regular review of any significant events or complaints, and also to elicit, and reflect on, feedback from patients and peers. Adequate evidence from all these activities will allow the appraiser to complete your Form 4 each year and provide the basis for the PCO to sign off the vast majority of GPs as not providing any cause for concern in terms of their fitness to practise. In this way it is hoped that the formative developmental role of appraisal can be maintained, whilst not requiring a duplicate set of information to be produced in order to revalidate each doctor.

PHCTs appraisal

Motivated and skilled staff are the key to delivering high-quality services to people needing health and social care. Staff working in primary care are committed to the personal and professional development of their staff, and believe that appraisal of staff is fundamental to the delivery of this vision. It is therefore expected that every employee will participate in the appraisal process. There are different models of delivering appraisal and so you wish to explore the most appropriate model for your particular GP practice before deciding which to adopt. The two main types of appraisals involve direct line manager appraisal and 360 degrees appraisal. Although there are different ways of delivering appraisals, the purpose and principles are the same.

Purpose of appraisal

The purpose of appraisal is to:
- **focus** on an individual's effort so that personal, professional and organisational objectives are met and overall performance is enhanced;
- **define** personal, professional and organisational objectives;
- **assess** progress towards the achievement of personal, professional and organisational objectives; and
- **identify** action required, including training and education interventions, to achieve objectives, to improve overall performance and to enhance motivation.

Principles of appraisal

The principles underlying the appraisal process are as follows:
- Appraisal is *developmental and motivational,* not punitive and not related to pay (unless stated in the contract of employment). Poor performance is dealt with in other policies and procedures. It is both a retrospective and prospective process that seeks to build on past achievements and to plan the year ahead.
- Appraisal is *two-way,* giving the employee as well as the manager the right to state views and propose courses of action.
- Every individual is *entitled to at least one appraisal discussion per year* but appraisal is regarded as an ongoing process with feedback and action points being discussed as and when appropriate throughout the

year. The appraisal discussion is a chance to consolidate and develop what is already known, not to introduce new issues that have never been raised before.

- The appraisal discussion is an *open and honest* conversation between two people and is *confidential* to them, apart from when the involvement of others is needed to effect agreed action points or where confidentiality would damage patient care or the corporate responsibilities of the employing GP practice or PCO.
- The *matters for discussion* in appraisal include the individual's career aspirations, work–life balance issues, professional development in terms of skills, knowledge and qualifications, service objectives, and corporate issues such as health and safety, risk management and governance.

Every individual will own a PDP that they themselves are responsible for maintaining and updating, assisted as far as possible by the GP practice or PCO.

Appraisal process

At least once a year the member of staff will meet with his or her line manager (and professional head if this is appropriate) to:

- review **achievements** of previously set personal, professional and organisational objectives;
- discuss personal, professional and organisational **aspirations** for the future;
- define specific personal, professional and organisational **objectives;** and
- identify **actions** to be taken to achieve the objectives.

Appraisal training

Regular training courses in appraisal are usually organised jointly by the GP practices and training departments of PCOs. All appraisers are expected to attend these courses so that the maximum benefit for all concerned can be achieved. Records of appraisals may vary between GP practices. The following model may be adopted or adapted to suit individual practice needs.

Preparing for appraisal

Prior to a formal appraisal meeting, the manager and appraisee should agree what documents/information the member of staff should bring to the meeting to assist with the process, depending on the role of the individual member of staff.

- To assist with the review of your performance and achievements, relevant documents may include:
  - Your job description and employee specification
  - Previously agreed team or individual objectives
  - Any other supporting information, e.g. in relation to projects or working groups that you have been involved with
- To assist with planning your objectives for the coming year, relevant documents may include:
  - Local delivery plan
  - Team or department objectives/business plan
  - Clinical governance plan
  - Clinical audit plan

Criteria for funding or other assistance

Many development needs can be met from a variety of sources that the individual or the individual's manager can access for himself/herself. These include job shadowing, guided reading, mentoring, secondment, and coaching.

Some will need to be met by attendance at courses either provided by the education and training departments of the respective organisation or by external providers. Where funding is required for courses, this may be accessed from a number of potential sources. Requests for funding for courses are usually directed in the first instance to the line manager.

Where funding or other assistance is required, priority will be given to statutory training (required by the law) or mandatory training (required by the PCO, County Council or the individual's professional body). In addition, there is training that is essential to maintain current standards and services and to support new developments.

Documentation

Documentation should be kept to a minimum but a record of key points should be made on the appraisal pro forma and placed on the personal file. Record of key points will include:

- achievements;
- aspirations;
- objectives, each supported by key results expected, actions required and timescales; and
- a personal and professional development plan. Training needs should be clearly identified, along with the agreed preferred method of meeting those needs. Where there are funding implications or other assistance is required from the respective education and training departments, Workforce Development Confederation or other external source, these costs will be clearly identified on the plan. A representative from the GP practice or PCO will usually meet once a year with representatives from the respective education and training departments to plan the delivery of the identified training needs, taking account of the training needs identified through appraisal.

The individual should also take a copy of their development plan to keep with themselves. It is further recommended that everyone should keep their own development folder containing the plan, plus evidence of achievement as it is collected throughout the year.

THE HEINZ MEDICAL PRACTICE: FORMAL RECORD OF STAFF APPRAISAL

Name	Ms A Praisal
Job title	Practice Manager
Place of work	The Heinz/Medical Practice
Length of time in this post	2 years 3 months
Name of appraiser	Dr R Songal
Date appraisal completed	9th June 2005

Review of performance and achievements

Factors that have helped you to fulfil your role and meet objectives (includes progress in meeting previously identified training and development needs)	Factors that have hindered you being able to meet the role outlined in your job description or objectives
1 Supportive management 2 Dedicated practice team 3 Appropriate admin support 4 Protected time and funding for continuing personal development 5 Supportive and challenging wider network (e.g. practice manager support group)	1 Significant organisational change 2 Significant budgetary limitations: restrictions on funding of practice manager conferences 3 Changing and differential expectations of and from clinical leads 4 Changing professional role 5 Multiple and competing demands of PCOs 6 Staffing changes

Other achievements over the last year
1 Production of practice manager education strategy in partnership with four other GP practices in locality. 2 Successful establishment of multi-agency clinical guidelines study group. 3 Successful establishment of partnerships with local RDSU for wider strategic links. 4 Assisted GP colleagues in two successful research bids for clinical trials into step-down treatment of beta-2 antagonists in asthma treatment. 5 Consolidated staffing in both primary care health teams: completed all annual appraisals of practice staff. 6 Developed and implemented new appraisal system and procedures within the practice. 7 Update courses in Basic Life Support, Performance management, and Powerpoint for future attendance at conferences. 8 Successfully passed all coursework components of my part-time Doctorate in Professional Practice.

Planning

Objective	Action required to achieve	By whom and due date	Notes on attainment (to be completed at following appraisal)
1 BLS update	Attend PCO conference	June 2005 (AP/RS)	
2 Establish practice business plan	Project work with practice manager	July 2005 (AP/RS)	
3 Establish practice skills mix matrix	Practice work with PHCT	Aug 2005 (AP/RS)	
4 Complete doctorate Year 4 (Thesis)	Continued work with academic supervisor	Dec 2005 (AP/RR)	

Personal development plan

Your hopes and aspirations for your career and work–life balance

Short-term plan (within next year)	Medium-term plan (2–5 years)	Long-term plan (over 5 years)
As above	Achieve wider responsibility for managing local HPE scheme for new GPs	Managing a larger community practice

Training and development needs

Training/development need	Preferred method of meeting this need	Priority	Costs (include course fees, travel, backfill)

Methods of meeting identified training needs may include:
- Shadowing/rotational opportunities
- Mentoring/buddying
- Self-directed learning
- Training courses or workshops

Priority:
1 = Statutory and/or mandatory training
2 = Essential to maintain current standards
3 = Necessary to support new developments
4 = Not directly relevant to current post

Summary and comments

To be completed by the appraisee

I am pleased with my progress over this past year and have achieved all of my work objectives which we agreed last year. I have enjoyed helping new staff settle into post and feel that I have developed a business approach to the management of the practice with the introduction of a new patient record system and staff appraisal process.

I look forward to meeting my agreed work objectives in the coming year.

Signed... Date................................

Summary and comments

To be completed by the appraiser

This has been an excellent year in which you have achieved all of your work objectives which we agreed last year. You have contributed effectively in many ways to the management of the practice and have helped new staff settle into post. I have been particularly pleased with the way you have prioritised and managed your increasing workload with a practical and positive approach to problem solving, working in a demanding and changing work environment. Well Done!

Signed... Date....................................

Summary and comments

To be completed by the appraisee

Signed... Date................................

Summary and comments

To be completed by the appraiser

Signed... Date....................................

360 degrees feedback
What is 360 degrees feedback?

The principle of using managers' feedback on an individuals' performance is an established process within the public and private sector. It is used to inform both performance management and appraisal discussions. However, over the last two decades businesses have been applying this process more widely employing what is termed the '360 degrees feedback' method of appraising individuals. In essence, think of the person being reviewed as being in the middle of a circle with peers responding with feedback from 90 degrees, other colleagues at 180 degrees, clients/external contacts at 270 degrees and superiors at 360 degrees. Thus, a 'full circle' of feedback is obtained.

In 360 degrees feedback the process used differs from traditional evaluations as the feedback comes from a **range of different sources,** which is accepted as being more balanced, fair and objective.

What are the benefits?

- Multiple sources of information tend to be more **objective** and **valid**.
- Comprehensive information about a GP can be sought on **multiple dimensions** in a **structured** way.
- Using 360 degrees feedback is a useful way to help GPs collect some of the less **easily accessible** information required for GMC revalidation (e.g. evidence of effective relationships with colleagues and patients).
- It can both help individuals understand how others perceive them and help them consider negative feedback in a positive, constructive and less defensive way.
- Feedback can be motivating and help focus GP's personal and professional development activities, which ultimately improves patient care.
- When everyone in a practice uses 360 degrees feedback it often results in better communication between team members and strengthens team working.

What format does 360 degrees feedback take in the health service?

The GMC is interested in the use of 360 degrees feedback as a tool to inform personal reflection and development as part of the appraisal process, and to assist with data collection for revalidation. This tool is not new within the NHS. Different methods include using open-ended unstructured interviews, statements with simple rating scales and structured questionnaires based upon items from focus groups with GPs and consultants.

It would seem likely that in future the use of 360 degrees feedback will become more widespread across the NHS, especially as part of GP's revalidation process. There are existing tools specifically developed for this purpose (see over the page for further details).

What evidence is there that 360 degrees feedback is helpful for doctors?

Research from the United States suggests that valid feedback on GP's performance can be effectively obtained by seeking structured feedback from a minimum of 11 peers (Ramsey *et al.* 1993). These findings showed that the feedback results were not influenced by the GP–peer relationship or the method used.

What do you need to be aware of when implementing the process?

The implementation of 360 feedbacks appraisal is much easier and potentially effective in a supportive, developmental culture. For this reason it is helpful if those 'at the top' take part in the process first to set the scene for other members of the organisation. If a GP practice wants to implement the process, it is important that the partners demonstrate a willingness to engage in the process in order to create a supportive, non-threatening culture for all members of the team. We should not underestimate the power of this!

One point of note: 360 degrees appraisal methods will clearly *not* work in dysfunctional practices. The culture and working atmosphere needs to be sufficiently open and secure to deal with colleagues making comments about each other.

Individuals being appraised are less likely to feel threatened by the feedback if they themselves can select the colleagues and contacts by whom they wish to get the questionnaire completed.

Respondents need a clear briefing including the following points, so they understand why the process is taking place:

- The process is aimed at helping the individual doctor's development.
- The appraisee has selected them specifically to provide structured feedback.
- The results will be anonymous (this is important as they may wish to say something which could appear negative).
- An external agency/person will collate the results and the individual doctor will only see the anonymised final report – so no individuals giving feedback are identifiable.

Currently feedback from patients is sought via separate patient surveys, mainly because the specific issues focused on will be different for colleagues and patients. To get a comprehensive picture of how you are perceived by others at work you need to obtain feedback from both patients (via a patient survey) and colleagues (via the 360 degrees process) and look at the results of these together. The appraisal discussion provides an ideal forum for this.

What tools are available to doctors?

An Internet search will show that a wide range of consultancies offer 360 degrees feedback surveys. Many will design questionnaires for use by your specific practice/department; however, the cost will vary. You always need to check that the tool is well validated and easy to administer and interpret.

There have also been 360 degrees services specifically developed for doctors. The authors of this article are specifically aware of two such examples:

- CFEP, an organisation based at Exeter University, has developed the *Colleague Feedback Evaluation Tool*, which is well validated and available for both GPs and consultants. They also offer a patient survey service (contact Tel. 01392 252740).
- Edgecumbe Consulting Group, based in Bristol, has developed the *Doctors Insight 360*, which is a confidential 360 degrees feedback service and has been used successfully by many GPs and consultants (contact Tel. 0117 925 8822).

GPs have been directly involved in developing both of the above tools and therefore they have been developed with an understanding of the environments within which they will be used.

Potential disadvantages
- Some 360 degree tools are more robust and valid than others.
- There will generally be a degree of non-response to the survey.
- Some respondents may not be completely honest for fear of identification, even when anonymity is guaranteed.
- The feedback is still taken only from a sample of individuals and so can never be taken as wholly representative.

How to link results with appraisal and revalidation effectively?
360 degrees feedback should be used for **developmental** purposes only (and *not* performance management). Thus, the final feedback report should go directly to the individual doctor concerned for him/her to pass on to his or her appraiser. He or she will then have the chance to read and reflect upon the feedback and think about his or her personal development needs.

By discussing the feedback report with his/her appraiser, he/she can be helped to identify strengths that can be maximised and used to maintain good medical practice and development needs to put into his/her PDP. Further, the 360 degrees feedback results should not be taken as stand-alone evidence of a doctors' performance. Other evidence must be considered and discussed to enable the appraiser and appraisee to identify overall patterns and themes. The discussion of the report and other evidence should be wholly developmental and well supported.

The final feedback report can then go into the revalidation documentation folder as part of the evidence that the GP has validly reflected upon aspects of their practice including relationships with colleagues and patients, and taken supported steps to act upon the report's findings.

In summary
360 degrees feedback is here to stay, and experience shows that it can be a very effective personal development tool if well selected and fed back in a developmental and supportive way.

360 degrees feedback picks up on behaviours that are core to good clinical skills and can help determine a GP's ability to provide effective, caring and compassionate care. The opportunity to collect comprehensive data to help reflect upon and refine these skills is a valuable one.

One final thought: Emotional competence is one of the most important components of a successful career, and self-awareness is the key element in this. It is therefore vital that we become aware of our own 'blind spots' and consider how these may impact on others.

Useful websites for *Appraisal*

DoH site for general information about appraisal and electronic versions of all the forms — www.doh.gov.uk/gpappraisal/index.htm

DoH sponsored SCHIN site which was set up to guide GPs through their data collection for appraisal and to fill in and store all their appraisal forms online – easy to access and lots of useful tips — www.appraisals.nhs.uk

New BMJ site which guides you through the production of your PDP and the ongoing collection of data – easy to use and many useful links — www.bmjlearning.com

Information on appraisal and revalidation — www.appraisaluk.info

GMC website with up-to-date information on appraisal and revalidation — www.gmc-uk.org

RCGP website – ongoing debate about revalidation also has the GP version of Good Medical Practice — www.rcgp.org.uk

An educational package using web-based technology to help develop skills in appraisal — www.appraisal-skills.com

A joint DoH and GMC website designed as a support tool to guide and assist doctors throughout the process of appraisal and revalidation — www.revalidationuk.info

A support website for GP appraisers – — www.gpappraisal.nhs.uk

Other useful websites

The Shipman Enquiry — www.the-shipman-inquiry.org.uk

National Association of Primary Care Educators — www.napce.net

Edgecumbe Consulting – 360 degrees — www.edgecumbe.com/edge/

Client-Focused Evaluations Program (CFEP) — www.cfep.net/

A full list of websites can be found on pages 192–197.

Audit and research

Research and development (R & D) in primary care

Research is exciting and rewarding, and is fundamental to the health sciences. Historically, the epidemiological research undertaken by GPs has made a significant contribution to the health of the nation, for example the aetiology and eradication of smallpox; the causes of yellow fever and typhoid fever; the epidemiology of heart disease; and the spread of infection in infectious hepatitis.

Interested and enthusiastic individual practitioners can do important research. However, some research questions are difficult to answer by one GP on his/her own, and may require a much larger population base than that within one practice. A team approach, with the active involvement of a number of participating practices, opens up more research opportunities and the potential for the pooling of expertise. One way of linking with other GPs with research interests is through the primary care research networks.

Although most NHS contacts occur and end in general practice, currently only a small proportion of clinical research involves general practice. There are many reasons for this, not least the lack of time and space in most surgeries. However, other barriers such as the lack of availability of research training, academic support, and research funding can now be overcome. The research networks can provide help and information. The NHS Executive provides expert advice and assistance to all health care professionals on the design and conduct of R&D projects, in both the primary and secondary care sectors.

Perhaps you are not so keen on undertaking or participating in original research, but are concerned that your health care decisions should be based on best research evidence, not opinion or guesswork! There are courses that focus on the sources of evidence and how to find them, as well as on how to critically appraise research findings. The research networks can provide you with appropriate information.

Undertaking research, finding relevant literature, and appraising it are only part of the process of evidence-based practice. The other two components relate to deriving the important questions in the first place and, at the other extreme, applying the results.

As far as the former is concerned, questions are most often initiated within a specific patient encounter. Please let the research community know where the gaps in research are and what should be the priorities for further research. Calls for applications for research funding in these areas are then likely to be initiated.

Finally, GPs make important health care decisions within the unique patient-practitioner consultation. This points to the importance of practitioners being up to date and knowing what is best evidence. Please take advantage of some of the help that is available. You will then have the flexibility to use the evidence within the patient consultation, taking into account the situation and preferences of a specific patient.

Using evidence in the management of common diseases

Evidence-based medicine is the term used to describe the application of research evidence into everyday medical practice. It has been defined as:

> The process of systematically reviewing, appraising and using clinical research findings to aid the delivery of optimum clinical care to patients. (Davidoff 1999)

The development and promotion of the concept of evidence-based practice achieved prominence in the 1990s with authors such as Sackett *et al.* (1997).

Using hard, objective, scientific evidence from investigations typified by the double-blind randomised controlled trial to assess the effectiveness or otherwise of medical interventions is hard to challenge on common-sense grounds alone; indeed how could anyone argue against something so obviously correct as basing our practice on objective evidence?

Evidence can be ranked in descending order of credibility:

- Strong evidence from at least one systematic review of multiple well-designed randomised controlled clinical trials.
- Strong evidence from at least one properly designed randomised controlled trial of appropriate size.
- Evidence from well-designed trials such as non-randomised trials, cohort studies, time series or matched case-controlled studies.
- Evidence from well-designed non-experimental studies from more than one centre or research group.
- Opinions of respected authorities, based on clinical evidence, descriptive studies or reports of expert committees.

Nevertheless, authors such as Davidoff (1999) point out that there are other factors that dictate our choice of action as the following diagram illustrates.

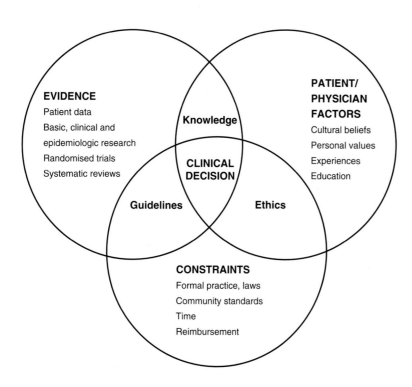

Humans are unique individuals whose responses vary idiosyncratically and biologically, and can be diluted or lost through the statistical treatment of data. Variation in age, sex and the presence of multiple pathologies can interfere with the interpretation and application and findings. In addition, the cookbook approach that this philosophy might be seen as advocating does not take into account individual patients' contraindications to treatment, volition, understanding and compliance with recommendations. Critics also argue that aspects such as economic, ethical, psychological, contextual and organisational issues must in addition be brought into the decision-making equation.

However, research can tell us which medical interventions really do work and which do not. Perhaps we are all guilty to a greater or lesser extent of practising medicine in a way that we have always done or we ignore evidence, e.g. prescribing antibiotics for viral infections. Most of us find it difficult to change the habits of a lifetime or are susceptible to patient pressure.

The aim of evidence-based medicine is to ensure that clinical decisions are backed by the evidence of what is and what is not effective treatment, e.g. prescribing aspirin for the secondary prevention of coronary heart disease. Our skills as professionals is to use our professional judgement to offer what we believe to be the most appropriate plan of action in each individual circumstance.

Reasons given for avoiding changing practice have been identified as scepticism, information overload and lack of time, skills, resources and motivation (Wilkinson *et al.* 1999).

Evidence of various sorts is now so plentiful that the way it is selected is important. The origin of the evidence is hugely important and the bias it has must be considered. Finding the best evidence is not always easy. Local medical libraries can help and will undertake literature searches. Use of the Internet is the most common and a route into a medically orientated search facility is now available to all practices. Use of familiar and favourite websites is also helpful, as long as you are aware of any bias they may have.

To select evidence to use and to apply it requires several steps:

- Ask the right questions.
- Access information.

Journal clubs	Each team member presents an original paper and comments upon it. Critical review of original papers is an important part of setting the findings into a local context.	Bias from individual members preferences and experience.
Use of databases, e.g. Cochrane	There are many databases now available to all NHS clinicians. These provide reviews of studies in similar areas and usually give a commentary that can provide an accumulation of current academic thinking.	Bias from expert's point of view, and from availability of evidence.
National guidance	NICE, NSFs and the nGMS provide very specific recommendations.	Bias from national pressures and political requirements.
Local care pathways	These often provide a good source of understanding how the local health community tackles problems.	Bias from local habits and availability of care.
Soft evidence	Clinical experience, patient feedback and local knowledge are all valid types of evidence.	Bias from individual experience.

? Do any of these barriers to changing practice apply to you?

- Appraise and critically evaluate the evidence.
- Apply the evidence to your own situation.
- Assess the effects of change.
- Audit.

In order to understand the evidence and to use it effectively there are a number of ways a practice can look at it. Each approach has its own bias.

Clinical governance is about the appropriate selection of evidence, sharing discussion of it, and using it wisely. In many ways it could be said to be more important for members of the practice to all take part in the formation of local clinical pathways and formularies by using the evidence to create them than it is for them all to follow other people's guidance.

Learning in groups – an example

To help people make sense of evidence about effectiveness, the former Oxford Regional Health Authority set up the Critical Appraisal Skills Programme (CASP). In developing methods of helping people appraise reviews of evidence, CASP has worked closely with the UK Cochrane Centre and the McMaster University of Canada.

The CASP team, based in Oxford, holds training sessions. The workshop format is constantly evaluated and improved. There is a talk on clinical effectiveness, including types of trials, reviews, and meta-analysis, together with some basic definitions of epidemiological and statistical terms. Participants then work in small groups to solve a problem scenario, such as whether or not dyspeptic patients who are positive for *Helicobacter pylori* should be treated with triple therapy. The problem is tackled by critically appraising an article about the clinical effectiveness of that problem.

Different participants will get different things from a CASP workshop. Some people only require an awareness of the importance of finding and appraising evidence, others will actually want to acquire the skills of critically appraising evidence, and a few will require the skills to enable them to write literature reviews.

Learning yourself

To find out which treatment works and which does not, you may wish to seek advice from your local medical librarian or you can look at the literature yourself.

The following list of publications may be helpful:

British Medical Journal	*Evidence Based Purchasing*
Lancet	*Evidence Based Medicine*
British Journal of General Practice	*Journal of Evidence Based Medicine*
Family Practice	*Drugs and Therapeutics Bulletin*
Bandolier	*Effective Health Care*
MeReC Bulletins	*Education for Primary Care*

However, the development of the Internet and electronic databases has revolutionised ability to access information, and a list of useful websites can be found on page 192. This has also influenced relationships with patients, who can just as easily search for information. This, while sometimes challenging in the consultation, can enhance quality of care, although issues of quality and commercial interest need to be taken into account.

USING EVIDENCE IN THE MANAGEMENT OF COMMON DISEASES

Clinical problem

Secondary prevention of CHD

EXAMPLE

Is there any evidence about which treatment works and which does not?

- Physical activity – British Regional Heart Study
- Diet (recent BHS Information sheet for references)
- Stop smoking
- Aspirin – ISIS2 study
- BP control – Hypertension optimal treatment study
- SMAC guidelines

How would I find out about the most effective treatment?

- Medline and Cochrane Database
- University of York's 'Effective Health Care'
- Guidelines publication
- Drugs and Therapeutics Bulletin

USING EVIDENCE IN THE MANAGEMENT OF COMMON DISEASES

Clinical problem

Is there any evidence about which treatment work and which does not?

How would I find out about the most effective treatment?

Practice audit

There is now widespread recognition that a completed audit cycle is the educational vehicle for learning about change. For a variety of reasons, however, it can be very difficult to implement. A key issue is good preparation and a firm structure linked to a practical issue. A suggested format could be the following:

- Define the precise area of care to be audited.
- Prepare and plan involving all key members of the practice.
- Review criteria defined and standards set.
- Define a time for data collection.
- Analyse data against the standards set.
- Feed back data to the practice with agreement on change to be implemented and date for evaluation of change.

The crucial issue is that responsibility should be taken by an individual member of the practice (probably the manager) to oversee the audit within the practice. One suggestion is for the practice to develop an audit calendar for the year with specific areas being audited in specific months or quarters.

Example of an administrative audit

Title of Audit. Registration of newborn babies in the practice.

Criterion. Newborn babies in the practice should be registered within 6 weeks.

Standard Set. Ninety-five per cent of babies will have completed registration forms by 6 weeks from birth.

Preparation and Planning. The practice manager had been aware that the practice was missing out on newborn baby registrations because of the lack of a system for ensuring they were properly registered with the practice. He/she called a meeting of the partners, the health visitors and the practice nurse, and they decided to check the registration details over the last 6 months. The health visitor was delegated to collect the numbers of babies born in the practice over this time and the manager checked the date of birth and date of registration.

Data Collection (1). Thirty babies born with 20 registered at 6 weeks (66%).

Change to be Implemented. A simple pro forma was drawn up with the headings: name of baby, date of birth and date registered. This was to be put in every patient's antenatal file and completed by the 6-week postnatal check.

Data Collection (2). This was carried out 6 months later. Forty babies born, 36 babies registered at 6 weeks (90%).

Conclusion. A simple tracking mechanism is usually necessary to ensure that patients do not fall through the system with consequent lack of follow-up and potential loss of income. Newborn babies are often at risk of this, particularly in families where there are more pressures, such as the disadvantaged. A team effort and a tight protocol, simply kept, can ensure that these risks are minimised.

Example of a practice audit

A 65-year-old man arrives in the surgery with a proven bladder tumour. You note that microscopic haematuria had been recorded by the nurse 3 months previously but not followed up by the doctor, raising the possibility that the tumour could have been diagnosed earlier.

A significant-event analysis is carried out within the practice and it is further noted that there is no procedure for following up urine specimens sent to the laboratory. The practice decided that 95% of laboratory urine specimens should have a recorded follow-up in the records. A retrospective search through the case records over the past 4 weeks of laboratory urine specimens showed that 45% had a follow-up urine result in the records. All laboratory urine specimens were recorded in a book held by reception staff and a further column was added, which was then ticked when the follow-up sample was recorded. Gaps could then be easily identified and followed up. Three months later a repeat collection of data over a similar period was carried out and the percentage of laboratory urine specimens followed up had risen to 88%.

Lessons learned were that a simple change in the recording method allowed easy follow-up and, in particular, identification of defaulters. Costs were saved by defining those specimen samples that should be tested in the practice and those that should be sent to a laboratory. Suboptimal care was rectified by improved follow-up and management.

After reading the above audits you may wish to tick the box if you felt that the criterion was present.

Criterion   Present

Reason for choice of audit	Potential for change Relevant to the practice	☐
Criterion/criteria chosen	Relevant to audit subject and justifiable (e.g. current literature)	☐
Standards set	Targets towards a standard with a suitable timescale	☐
Preparation and planning	Evidence of teamwork and adequate discussion where appropriate	☐
Data collection (1)	Results compared against standard	☐
Change(s) to be evaluated	Actual example described	☐
Data collection (2)	Comparison with Data collection (1) and standard	☐
Conclusions	Summary of main issues learned	☐

 Would you like to add this to your PPDP and individual PDPs?

Significant-event auditing (SEA)

While looking at groups of patients can give powerful insights into care, it can be difficult to turn discussion into action. It is common for repeat conventional audits to show little change for the better. However, we often dramatically change our behaviour when something happens to one patient: for example, a patient is registered partially sighted as a result of diabetic retinopathy, and we carry out fundoscopy with renewed enthusiasm.

Significant-event auditing is a method for harnessing the intellectual rigour of conventional audit to the emotional drive of 'adverse events'. It can therefore be:

- enjoyable (we all like discussing clinical cases);
- stimulating (it is *our* management of the patient that is being discussed!);
- evidence based (no wild decisions, but well-organised outcomes); and
- productive (decisions stick and care is improved).

  The benefits of SEA are clear in terms of clinical governance, improving quality of patient care and learning. SEA now attracts points under QOF and additional points and funding can be awarded if the practice undertakes the following:
- A minimum of 6 SEAs in the past 3 years.
- A minimum of 12 SEAs in the past 3 years which include (if they have occurred):
  - Any death on practice premises
  - Two new cancer diagnoses
  - Two deaths involving terminal care
  - One patient complaint
  - One suicide
  - One section under the Mental Health Act.

The basic tenets

A group of significant cases is discussed, not only those where something has gone wrong, but also those that give insight into our care. The discussion is not intended to allocate blame, but to agree how, if at all, care can be improved. None of us is perfect and we need to learn from each other's imperfections. There are six possible outcomes from the discussion:

1 congratulations for care well given;
2 further investigation of the topic (search for evidence);
3 conventional audit;
4 immediate changes (only when justified);
5 identification of an educational need; and
6 decision that nothing needs to be done.

What is a significant event?

In short, it is anything that any member thinks notable, clinically or organisationally. Normally all MIs, infections, strokes, new cancers, unplanned pregnancies, attempted or successful suicides, osteoparotic fractures or acute visits for asthma, epilepsy or diabetes will be listed, as well as any patient complaint, administrative mix-up (visit requested but not carried out) or prescribing problem. Your practice may appoint a 'practice coordinator' to prompt primary health care teams to identify events, keep a record of discussion and actions and disseminate information.

To maximise the success of introducing SEA into your practice, it is useful to think about the best ways to make the process appealing to the team. To be successful the participants must feel comfortable, both physically and professionally. This includes appropriate timing, maybe even with sandwiches for a working lunch. A no-blame culture needs to be adopted from the outset and this needs pointing out to all concerned. Some teams may find it more appealing to begin with just the doctors, adding other members of the team as confidence grows and the process develops.

Careful selection of the first event is essential. It is best to start with something that, while being important, is not too emotive; a very difficult or serious problem may fracture the team before enough confidence has been developed and the method is trusted. This will give the team the strength it will need to tackle more testing events in the future.

After nearly 15 years' experience of SEA, it is generally believed to be the single-most powerful tool for improving care and identifying educational needs. For further details, it is recommended that you read 'Occasional Paper 70' from the Royal College of General Practitioners.

Ideas for subjects to use when thinking of significant events

- New cancer cases.
- Unplanned pregnancies.
- Sudden death.
- Trauma, suicide.
- Drug reaction.
- Terminal care.
- Patient complaints.
- Breach of confidentiality.
- Aggressive patients.
- Home visits not carried out.
- Rota and staffing problems.
- Communication problems.
- Appointment problems.
- Legal – anything about this.
- Prescribing or dispensing error.

RECORDING A SIGNIFICANT EVENT

	Action	Deadline
What happened? JP saw a Bath hospital employee who wanted a termination but not at her own hospital		
How did it affect: **The Patient** She wanted it to be carried out in Bristol to ensure confidentiality **You** Not sure how to go about referring Bath patients to Bristol **The practice** Also unsure about correct procedure for referral of patients to Bristol for termination of pregnancy		
Why did it happen? Not sure of the procedure/option		
Steps to be taken to avoid similar events in future: Contact the local pregnancy advisory service for details of Bristol consultants		
Learning needs revealed by the event: How to arrange termination out of the area for staff members, need efficient system to ensure patients seen quickly		
How will these be met? Contact the local pregnancy advisory service in Bristol for details of their service especially with regard to staff members	Dr A	5th June 2005

PERSONAL SEA

Date:

Describe what happened?

How did it affect the patient?

How did it affect you?

How did it affect the practice?

Could it have been avoided?

Can it be stopped from happening again?

What learning or development needs has this highlighted for you personally?

What learning or development needs has it highlighted for others?

HEINZ MEDICAL PRACTICE – RECORDING A SIGNIFICANT EVENT

Date of meeting	31st March 2005

Event	Questions	Action
A. Reported death of 66-year-old male asthmatic with COPD – died suddenly at home	Who else should be informed?	A. Has done bereavement visit today – family extends thanks to all at the surgery
B. Reported death of 96-year-old female – died of old age. Last seen 13 days ago	Any family?	No immediate family known
C. Received notification of death in hospital of female patient. Coroner's report requested as she did not recover from anaesthetic after operation for fracture	Any family?	No close relatives
C. Raised problem of staff shortages in reception	How long and what needs to be done to help?	B. Suggested district nurses could be asked to write out their prescription requests on blank scripts All GPs to be given their own repeat requests on a daily basis to print themselves. H. To coordinate
A. Reported new cancer. 56-year-old female seen by Sister X for breast examination. Known of lumps for a couple of months. Appointment made for last Thursday and scheduled for mastectomy at Hospital today	How can we advise patients to present early?	A. To write article for local paper B. To put article in newsletter C. To do notice board in waiting room
C. Reported on male patient following case conference today. Very suicidal but decision made not to section. BEWARE: patient has black belt in judo and selection of knives/swords. Past history of alcohol abuse. Adamant, does not want to be sectioned and will defend himself. Has withdrawn all contact with mental health team	Who else should be informed?	B. To notify Emergency Doctors' Service
B. Has had several patients recently who said they were not aware that they could see Dr F or Dr G instead of their registered GP	Should they be aware?	All patients were sent a letter clearly explaining the new system. Receptionists advise patients every day. B. To publicise in newsletter

RECORDING A SIGNIFICANT EVENT

Date of meeting

Event	Questions	Action

MINUTES OF SIGNIFICANT EVENT AUDIT MEETING – HEINZ MEDICAL PRACTICE

Date	1st February 2005
Present	Dr A
	Dr B
	Dr C
	Practice nurse D
	Community nurses E and F
	Health visitor G
	Practice manager H
Apologies	Partners I and J
	Practice nurses K and L

SIGNIFICANT EVENT 1

Vaccinations for minors

BL who is a minor aged 13, came in for vaccinations with a relative. Unknown to the nurse, the relative left the surgery before the vaccination was completed

Outcome

Immediate change – the practice manager to instruct reception staff to always make sure, if possible, that a minor is never left in the surgery alone. If this happens, they must inform the nurse in the surgery. Nurses to refuse to treat any minor if they know a relative is not present

SIGNIFICANT EVENT 2

Routine review of sudden unexpected deaths within the last 3 months

7.15 a.m. Sunday. Male patient aged 53 years collapsed at home. Wife reported sudden onset of acute chest pain, pale, sweating. Ambulance attended – patient taken to hospital admitted Coronary Care Unit. Died Sunday p.m. – diagnosis acute anterior MI

Discussion

Review of medical records. Patient registered with the practice 1998.

Leaves wife aged 43 years and two children aged 10 and 13. Registration medical in 2000 incomplete. Known to be a smoker, BP 170/95, overweight at 107 kg, advised to return for blood pressure check in 3 months. Last seen in November 2004 by locum and prescribed antibiotic for chesty cough

Following his death his widow said that his father also died suddenly of a heart attack in his early fifties and his brother had an MI in his forties. The patient has a number of risk factors for CHD and illustrated a potentially avoidable death

Possible interventions include

- A more thorough registration medical, including taking a family history
- Advice and support to stop smoking
- Advice about diet and exercise
- Monitoring and perhaps treatment of hypertension
- Cholesterol screening

Outcome

- Audit to determine the percentage of patients who had not had a registration medical within 12 months of joining the practice
- Redesign computer template to include weight, BMI, BP and smoking status, family history of CHD and stroke, cholesterol and advice about diet and exercise

Learning opportunities for PPDP and PDP

Practice to arrange an evening meeting to review the evidence of what is effective in the prevention of primary and secondary CHD

Referral data

Comparative referral data is rarely absolutely accurate since some referrals will be missed (such as those to distant hospitals or ones made urgently) and they are sometimes coded wrongly. However, much of it is reasonably reliable. In consideration of the above, it is important to think in terms of rates per thousand of the population, or even rates per thousand of a particular age group. It may also be relevant within a practice setting to look at rates of individual doctors per session worked, rather than absolute numbers of referrals. In this way legitimate comparisons can be made.

It is generally helpful to develop a practice spreadsheet for referrals. The larger the number, the more reliable the relative data will be, but beware of looking at data over too long a time as referral criteria and available services change quite frequently and will affect rates.

Practice Population Profile

Total	Gender	0–4	5–15	16–44	45–64	75–84	85+	Expected changes
	Male							
	Female							

Referral rates

Specialty	Number	Number per 1000 population	PCO average per 1000 population	Percentage variation
General surgery				
Urology				
Orthopaedics				
ENT				
Opthalmology				
Plastic surgery				
Pain clinic				
General medical				
Gastroenterology				
Haematology				
Cardiology				
Dermatology				
Respiratory medicine				
Nephrology				
Neurology				
Rheumatology				
Paediatrics				
Geriatrics				
Mental health				

Similar tables could be drawn up for emergency admissions and for referrals to diagnostic or therapy services.

There are many reasons for variation from the local norm. If it is not obvious why your practice varies, it will be worth asking further questions of yourselves. You may need to look at individual referrals for this or consider your own and other local referral pathways and check that your criteria match others. If they do not you have to ask if it is legitimate to have a discrepancy. It may be, but if it is not, your referral may be blocking someone else from getting timely treatment. It is often suggested that those who have studied particular specialties for long make more referrals than those who have not. What has not been shown is whether those referrals result in improved outcomes or whether they are just the result of being aware of rare conditions that rarely occur.

When analysing your data you need to be as objective as possible and be open to changing your way of doing things. If your practice is also responsible for the payment resulting from referrals, your decision will be open to scrutiny not only by the local PCO but under the Freedom of Information Act 2000 it will be open to anyone to see. It will be important to be able to have clear criteria for decisions made especially if your referrals rates are significantly lower than similar areas or if your rates show marked changes. Referral pathways may be useful for this. Your PCO and other local practices may well have examples you can use, and it is helpful if your plans and pathways are similar to others. If you feel that there are significant differences with what you do and what others do, these differences should be aired through the PCOs clinical governance group.

Example

A practice was found to have very high referrals to gynaecology when compared with other local practices. A first question to be asked was whether this was an effect caused by only some of the referring doctors or were the referral rates the same through the practice. When it was found to be similar for all the referring doctors, the PCO information department was asked for a breakdown by age range for their practice and those of others. It immediately became clear that the rates per thousand patients of each age group were similar to other practices and that the reason for a comparatively high referral rate was solely caused by the relative age structure of the practice population.

Prescribing analysis and cost (PACT) prescribing

PACT data are available as two types of reports: PACT Standard Report and PACT Catalogue prepared by the Prescription Pricing Authority (PPA). All GPs are provided on a quarterly basis, or monthly on request, with a PACT Standard Report that gives detailed information about their prescribing from prescriptions that patients have had dispensed. GP registrars can monitor their prescribing by marking the prescription form with a 'D' in red ink alongside the GP identification number to facilitate feedback. This system is available for GP registrars only.

You can use PACT information to examine prescribing habits and cost, develop a practice formulary and monitor compliance with it or a district or PCO-wide formulary. This is powerful information and enables us to compare our performance against our colleagues both locally, at practice and PCO level, and nationally.

The PACT Standard Report provides information on your 20 most expensive prescription medicines, dressings or appliances, the number of prescription items and average cost per prescription item prescribed over a 3-month period. Prescribing in your top 40 British National Formulary (BNF) sections is also shown and allows us to examine prescribing across a range of therapeutic areas. Prescribing by other health professionals, nurses and pharmacists as well as supplementary prescribers working within the practice or directly employed by the PCO are also included and their totals are shown on the back page of the report.

PACT Standard Reports also contain articles in the centre pages discussing national guidance, recent clinical trials and prescribing trends for specific therapeutic areas; related practice-specific prescribing data are also provided.

The PACT Catalogue provides complete details of prescribing for any time period between 1 and 24 consecutive months and can be ordered for individual GPs or for the practice. Catalogues are also available for practice nurses and supplementary prescribers who prescribe within a practice or on behalf of a practice (PCO-employed prescribers). The PPA has started to provide prescribing and financial information for practices electronically (ePFIP), which will allow speedier access to prescribing data and eventually replace paper reports.

PACT information gives us the opportunity to look critically and monitor our prescribing, to audit and perhaps institute changes, which can be formally adopted by the whole practice and written into the PPDP. It is also the starting point for PCO prescribing advisers to discuss prescribing – drug choice, cost and trends – during the annual practice visit. As part of the new contract, practices are asked to action three areas of prescribing and to demonstrate that review has taken place.

THE PRACTICE PRESCRIBING COSTS FOR THE LAST QUARTER

We are above/below the PCO equivalent by	↑ 5%

We are above/below the national equivalent by	↑ 5%

BNF Therapeutic group significant above/below PCO
Significantly above in antibiotics, CVS and CNS

The 10 most expensive drugs used in the practice are:

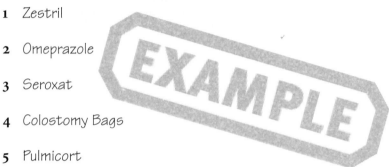

1   Zestril

2   Omeprazole

3   Seroxat

4   Colostomy Bags

5   Pulmicort

6   Simvastatin

7   Augmentin

8   Atorvastatin

9   Diclofenac

10   Losartan

The practice generic prescribing rate is above/below the PCO equivalent by	↑ 20%
Above/below the national equivalent by	↑ 10%
The practice generic prescribing rate is	65%
Has there been any significant change in the practice's PACT figures over the last 12 months?	YES
If YES, why has this change taken place? Increased generic prescribing rate by 20% and reduction in costs from 10% above primary care trust equivalent to 5%	
Do you plan to use this prescribing information to inform your PPDP?	YES
If YES, how? • To increase generic prescribing • To introduce a practice formulary	

THE PRACTICE PRESCRIBING COSTS FOR THE LAST QUARTER

We are above/below the PCO equivalent by

We are above/below the national equivalent by

BNF therapeutic group significant above/below PCO

The 10 most expensive drugs used in the practice are:

1

2

3

4

5

6

7

8

9

10

The practice generic prescribing rate is above/below the PCO equivalent by	
Above/below the national equivalent by	
The practice generic prescribing rate is	
Has there been any significant change in the practice's PACT figures over the last 12 months?	YES/NO
If YES, why has this change taken place?	
Do you plan to use this prescribing information to inform your PPDP?	YES/NO
If YES, how?	

Performance indicators – thinking beyond the numbers...

One of the key features of clinical governance, as discussed earlier (p. 17), is transparency. It is sometimes uncomfortable to think of your personal performance being subject to scrutiny but if you think of it from a patient's perspective they may not be expecting the best at all times but they are rightly expecting your care to be of an acceptable standard. The only way to really know how you are doing is to compare yourself to others. It is quite possible to claim that health care is tailored to the individual and that any statistical view is flawed. Taken in isolation, this is often true; however, collectively good information can tell us a great deal.

The introduction of the QOF in the nGMS provides a very good starting point for this exercise. You can see how your performance compares to a national standard and your PCO should be able to tell you how you compare with practices in your area. NSFs also provide benchmarks for performance – sometimes in different clinical areas or setting a higher standard – so do not overlook them!

However, to get the greatest benefit from any information, you need to look beyond the figures and ask yourself some more searching questions. For instance, see the following.

Why are we where we are?

Typically a PCO will provide a box plot to give a performance indicator. The following is an example of a typical box plot that the PCO might publish as a performance indicator (PI) to measure asthma care in practice.

The percentage of patients in a practice (>15 years old) who have a diagnosis of asthma:

Minimum		Maximum
5%	X	15%
	Your practice	

> **A** What does this PI tell you about this practice's diagnosis or management of asthma?
> **B** How might you use this information to improve this practice's care of asthmatics?

- The PI on its own tells us nothing about the clinical care of asthmatic patients. It does tell us that the recorded incidence of asthma is lower than most of the other local practices. This may be simply because it is not well recorded, because there really are fewer asthmatics or because some are not diagnosed.
- Further information is needed to understand the situation. If the rate of prescribing of inhaled steroids was looked at, it could be high, low or average. If it was average or high, a recording problem is possible or there may be a lot of patients with chronic obstructive pulmonary disease (COPD). How many of these have had spirometry? Does the prescribing need to be looked at in detail or do the diagnostic criteria for asthma and COPD that are being used need to be reviewed?

As a starting point, figures that are ±20% from the average or where you or your practice are in the top or bottom few of a PCO wide graph should be the areas to look at your rates. Equally, areas that you think may be different for you are worth particular consideration. You may find you are not as far out as you thought.

Where you find you have unexplained discrepancies the PCO information department may be able to provide more detailed information and some anonymous comparative information. There may not be a straightforward route to find this and information departments are always busy but questions asked through the clinical governance route are likely to get a favourable response.

When you are still left uncertain about what the figures really reveal, you can seek assistance from a number of sources. The first is the PCO information department. Another could be your pharmacy advisor and a third is the clinical governance group and, in particular, the clinical leads.

How might PIs be used to identify learning needs?

PIs might be produced to demonstrate how one organisation is performing or how that organisation compares with another. The organisation might be a PCO or practice, or indeed an individual GP.

---

1   What do you think is the purpose of PIs?

---

2   What are the advantages and disadvantages of commonly used PIs?

- HINT: Are PIs useful in simply informing or comparing? Do they bring about a change in behaviour? If so, how do they achieve this? Do most of them measure the most useful and relevant things to you – as a clinician – and your practice? If not, how might PIs be changed to measure something more useful? What would be useful?

---

3   How might PIs be improved?

---

4   Which of the currently available PIs do you think are relevant to bringing about a change in clinical behaviour?

---

5   Why did you identify these ones and not others?

Useful websites for *Audit and research*

Bandolier	www.jr2.ox.ac.uk/bandolier/
British Journal of General Practice	www.rcgp.org.uk/journal/
British Medical Journal	www.bmj.com/
British National Formulary	http://bnf.org/bnf/ www.corec.org.uk/
Centre for Evidence Based Medicine	www.cebm.net/
Clinical Audits – Options	www.nosa.org.uk/information/audit/ options.htm
Critical Appraisal Skills Programme (CASP)	www.phru.nhs.uk/casp/casp.htm
Data Protection Act 1998	www.hmso.gov.uk/acts/acts1998/ 19980029.htm
Drugs and Therapeutics Bulletin	www.dtb.org.uk/dtb/
Effective Health Care	www.rsmpress.co.uk/ehc.htm
Evidence Based Healthcare and Public Health	www.harcourt-international.com/ journals/ebhc/
Evidence Based Medicine	www.evidence-based-medicine.co.uk
Evidence Based Purchasing	www.jr2.ox.ac.uk/bandolier/band11/ b11-7
Freedom of Information Act 2000	http://www.foi-uk.org/about_foi.html www.jfponline.com/default.asp
Journal of Family Practice	
King's Fund	www.kingsfund.org.uk
Lancet	www.thelancet.com/
McMasters University Canada	www.mcmaster.ca/
Medical Research Council	www.mrc.ac.uk
Medicines and Healthcare Products Regulatory Agency	www.mhra.gov.uk
Medline	www.nlm.nih.gov
Mental Health Act 1983	www.dh.gov.uk/PublicationsAnd Statistics/Legislation/ActsAndBills/
National Patient Safety Agency	www.npsa.nhs.uk www.npcrdc.man.ac.uk
National Primary Care Research and Development Centre	
National Treatment Agency (Substance Misuse)	http://www.nta.nhs.uk/ www.york.ac.uk/inst/crd
NHS Centre for Reviews and Dissemination (CRD)	
Nurse Prescribing	
Patient Support Group leaflets	www.doh.gov.uk/nurseprescribing
Pharmaceutical Industry Competitiveness Taskforce	www.patient.co.uk http://www.advisorybodies.doh.gov. uk/pictf/
Prescription Pricing Authority	www.ppa.nhs.uk
Primary Care Research Network	www.ukf-pcrn.org
Research and Development Networks in the NHS	http://www.rdforum.nhs.uk/

A full list of websites can be found on pages 192–197.

The practice professional development plan (PPDP)

The PPDP is the central document by which the practice collates information about its activity and aspirations. The main *purpose* of the plan is to enable the PHCT to focus on the objectives and priorities for future years and to identify continuing needs.

The PPDP is first and foremost for the practice, and the *process* of producing the plan is as important as the final document. The production of the plan should involve all PHCT members.

The headings discussed in this workbook are given over the page as part of the review process, but there will, of course, be other subjects that are not covered, such as premises, IT, cooperatives, etc.

The plan will form an important *link* with the PCO and ensures that it is aware of your plans and development needs. It will also enable you to demonstrate your achievements in line with national and local priorities.

Components of the plan

The main components of the PPDP are detailed in the first column of the table given below.

> - Start by reviewing the previous year's objectives – were they actived?
> - Then use the list on the following pages to bring forward anything from the individual sections from this workbook, which you have identified as being suitable to add to your PPDP

PRACTICE PROFESSIONAL DEVELOPMENT PLAN – THE HEINZ MEDICAL PRACTICE

Mission Statement: To provide a comprehensive, friendly, professional and personal service, with time to discuss our patients' health care concerns

Components of PPDP	Key objectives (previous year)	Evidence of achievement? if yes – please give date	If not – why not?	Practice objective to be added to PPDP for this year	How are we going to achieve this?	By whom?	By when?
Local delivery plan	To ensure quality of access to health care services for entire practice population	Audit of attendance at practice by socio-economic and ethnic groups. Achieved June 05	N/A	Continue audit on annual basis	Produce audit schedule and continue to monitor attendance at practice of socio-economic and ethnic groups	Audit manager	Nov 05
Health needs assessment	To produce a comprehensive health needs assessment of local practice population, consistent with NSF priorities	Production of health needs assessment in partnership with PCO	N/A	Continue to liaise with PCO	Attendance at PCO meetings where HNA are discussed	Dr A	Ongoing
Practice SCOT analysis	To undertake a SCOT analysis for whole practice team	NO	Due to long-term staff sickness, meetings had to be postponed until later this year	Production of a whole team practice SCOT analysis together with recommenda-tions for changing practice	Establish schedule of dates for meetings, ensuring locum cover and facilitators are available	PM	31 March 2006
GP appraisal	This is a new government initiative	NO	Postpone-ment of launch of GP revalidation	Continue with existing peer appraisal of all partners	Book sessions and ensure locum cover available	PM	31 March 2006

The above examples should enable you to continue and complete your PPDP on the following pages!

PRACTICE PROFESSIONAL DEVELOPMENT PLAN – THE HEINZ MEDICAL PRACTICE

Mission Statement: To provide a comprehensive, friendly, professional and personal service, with time to discuss our patients health care concerns

Components of PPDP	Key objectives (previous year)	Evidence of achievement? if yes – please give date	If not – why not?	Practice objective to be added to PPDP for this year	How are we going to achieve this?	By whom?	By when?
Local delivery plan							
Health needs assessment							
Profile of practice population							
Key features of practice population							
Identification of top health problems in the practice							
Prioritising the list							
Planning interventions							
New priorities							
The primary health care team							
Practice SCOT analysis							
Learning styles of primary							

PRACTICE PROFESSIONAL DEVELOPMENT PLAN – THE HEINZ MEDICAL PRACTICE

Mission Statement: To provide a comprehensive, friendly, professional and personal service, with time to discuss our patients health care concerns

Components of PPDP	Key objectives (previous year)	Evidence of achievement? if yes – please give date	If not – why not?	Practice objective to be added to PPDP for this year	How are we going to achieve this?	By whom?	By when?
Health care team							
Skill mix of primary health care team							
GP appraisal							
Staff appraisal							
Using evidence in the management of common diseases							
Practice audit							
Significant event auditing							
Referral data							
PACT prescribing							
Performance indicators							

PART 3

Personal development plan

Framework for personal development plans (PDP)

PDPs will continue to play an important part in appraisal, clinical governance and 5-yearly revalidation. Your PDP is confidential, and should another person, such as your GP tutor or line manager see it for revalidation and/or appraisal purposes, you may ask him/her to sign a copy of the Confidential Declaration form (see p. 191).

A PDP looks at where you wish to be, for example, in the next 5 years: how you will achieve it, what resources you will need and what barriers you will meet.

This section introduces some methods and tools for developing a plan. Many of these will be familiar to GP trainers and recent GP registrars.

Whichever methods you choose, a simple process is outlined below which may be of help to you in structuring your learning and deciding what could go into your portfolio.

Getting started

We suggest you set aside protected time for this exercise. PHCT members have busy lives, and it is easy to keep on working without making time to reflect. You can start by reflecting on your past achievements and goals for the future. The guides below can be used to help you move on and develop your PDP.

A **past educational profile** involves writing down all the educational positions and achievements of your career. A recent curriculum vitae will provide much of this information. You can list your specific educational highlights and achievements. An example of a past educational profile and pro forma can be found on page 138.

The **learning highlights** of the past few years is a simpler method that focuses on specific educational events or workshops that made a real impression on you. You might have learned a new skill, such as joint injections, gained managerial experience, or perhaps learned a new language! An example of how to record your learning highlights and pro-forma are on page 140.

A **self-audit** looks at your current situation and where you would like to go. A mentor or partner can augment this process considerably. It includes a personal **SCOT analysis** (see p. 142), listing your strengths and the challenges, identifying the opportunities for improvement or career progression and noting any threats to such progress.

When you have accomplished the above, you may have identified some major and minor areas of learning and development needs that you may wish to add to your PDP.

PAST EDUCATIONAL PROFILE

Position	Achievement
Associate GP tutor	Organising educational events Member of GP tutor group Liaison with PCO and Deanery
Advanced GP trainer's course	Remedial GP training Alternative educational approaches Importance of structure in GP training
Practice prescribing lead	Member of clinical governance group
Member of local Research Ethics Committee	Understanding ethics and research
Appraisal lead	Completing all practice appraisals on schedule

Does this highlight any gaps and objectives for the future?

Gaps	Future objectives
Small group leader training	Further develop my small group skills
Lack of clinical focus	Set up practice-based journal club
Clinical governance	Develop practice based multiprofessional learning
IT	Look for appropriate course to attend

PAST EDUCATIONAL PROFILE

Position	Achievement

Does this highlight any gaps and objectives for the future?

Gaps	Future objectives

LEARNING HIGHLIGHTS

The **learning highlights** of the past few years is a simpler method which focuses on specific educational events or workshops that made a real impression on you. You might have learned a new skill like joint injections, travelled or learned a new language or gained managerial experience. How was this event memorable for you and how did it influence your practice?

Key dates	What did you do?	Why?	What did you learn from this?	How have you used this?
August 2003	Sports Medicine Course	Large student population	Pathophysiology of injury: management of recovery	More appropriate management and use of secondary care
March 2004	Palliative Care Course	Elderly population Prevalence of chronic disease	Skills and attitudes relevant to terminal care	Continues to be used regularly
June 2004	Sexual Disease Screening Course	Increased incidence of STDs		The information provision to patients presenting with STDs
October 2004	Appraisal Training	New DoH guidance	Learned the importance of documenting achievements	Keeping my PDP more up to date
February 2005	Drug and Alcohol Dependency Course	A large number of drug- and alcohol-dependent patients	A wider range of different treatment options	The information provision to patients presenting with drug and alcohol dependency.
June 2005	Undertook a 6-week refresher evening course in conversational French	Wanted to go on holiday in France with my family	Learned enough to be able to get by on holiday and found that I had remembered much of my school French	Apart from enjoying our holiday, I would like to continue studying it in more depth and become sufficiently fluent

LEARNING HIGHLIGHTS

The **learning highlights** of the past few years is a simpler method that focuses on specific educational events or workshops that made a real impression on you. You might have learned a new skill like joint injections, travelled or learned a new language or gained managerial experience. How was this event memorable for you and how did it influence your practice?

Key dates	What did you do?	Why?	What did you learn from this?	How have you used this?

The self-audit and personal SCOT analysis

It is worth standing back occasionally and looking at who we are, where we are and where we would like to get to. Some people do this at regular intervals, such as birthdays or the start of the year. This has much to recommend it. Whenever it is done, the results can form the basis for rational objective setting, decision-making, planning and action.

Whatever the reason for undertaking a self-audit and personal SCOT analysis, it will always be necessary to be systematic, thorough and objective. This calls for a methodical framework and, if possible, input from at least one other person: a partner, close colleague, mentor, older child, friend or counsellor.

It is always best to work on paper. Some people find a large format such as flip chart or white board particularly helpful, especially if working with another person. Brainstorm each heading, listing as many possibilities as you can. Look back, refining and editing what you have written, and produce a final, polished listing you can keep and use.

The following checklists may help in the process, although the questions are not by any means exhaustive.

Ask yourself:

What qualifications have I got?

What special knowledge and experience have I got?

What support do I have from family and friends?

In so far as I have succeeded, what has helped me to do so?

What are the sources of my motivation and drive?

Have I any strong, specific interests, at work or outside?

Strengths and challenges are things that exist for you now. Opportunities and threats are possibilities that may come along in the future, but that need to be thought about now. You will need to maximise your strengths and opportunities and minimise your challenges and threats.

? Does this highlight any areas that should be added to your PDP?

My strengths
(relate to achievements over the year)

My challenges
(highlight any difficulties or obstacles that have been experienced)

My opportunities
(list factors that will influence your success, i.e. ideas for the future)

My threats
(obstacles to developing)

Methods of identifying educational needs

Sticky moments

This is a system that operates by identifying when a problem arising during a consultation is not met because of inadequate skills or knowledge. From this can be deduced what you need to learn so that next time you will be better equipped to deal with the problem.

The consultation is the pivotal transaction in general practice and it is during the consultation that one should start to identify learning needs by exploring whether a patient's need has been met. It is important to separate a patient's wants from a patient's needs (they may want a pill for their headache but need to come to terms with an unhappy marriage). It is easy to find out what you want to learn but much more of a challenge to identify their needs.

How is it done?

After each consultation, ask yourself 'Was I equipped to meet the patient's needs?'

To answer this question you must home in on the crux of the consultation and ask yourself whether you had the skills and knowledge to deal with it appropriately. You will soon find your first 'sticky moment'. At this point you must decide which category you are dealing with.

Is it:

Clinical knowledge	CK
Non-clinical knowledge	NCK
Skill	S
Attitude	A
Practice organisation	PO

Recording the 'sticky moment' and identifying educational and professional development needs

It is vital that the whole educational process is linked to improving patient care and remains relevant to everyday practice. Try and relate your education needs to a particular clinical situation. Record it on the 'Sticky moments' pro forma (see p. 146), which is totally confidential to you. Keep a copy of this pro forma on your desk so that you are able to record a 'sticky moment' as and when it arises. The process is as follows:

- Make a note of the consultation and the patient ID.
- Describe the sticky moment.
- Identify the educational need.
- Define area for improvement, development or change.
- Classify into category

- Decide how you are going to meet this need, for example you could:
  - Ask a colleague
  - Look it up in a textbook
  - Medline search
  - Journal club
  - Practice meetings.
- You may wish to use the Reflective Practice form on page 51 to describe what you have learned and how it may change your clinical behaviour.
- Collect the evidence of what you have learned in your portfolio.

In addition to an individual GP's 'sticky moments', there may be others which apply to the whole practice. (This is an excellent way of identifying significant events; see p. 114.)

Practice sticky moments and subsequent development needs may:

- support an individual needs;
- conflict with individual needs; and
- be irrelevant.

Try to provide at least one example of such an educational need in each category.

Supporting needs	Conflicting needs	Irrelevant needs

- Do you need to do anything as a result?
- Would you like to add this to your PDP?

Select one example of conflicting needs from above. How might this apparent tension in 'needs' be constructively resolved (a GP wishing to take an MSc course that does not form part of the practice plans)?

DISCOVERY PAGE – STICKY MOMENTS

Key:

Knowledge clinical	KC
Knowledge non-clinical	KNC
Skills	S
Attitude	A
Practice organisation	PO

Date	Patient Age	Sex	The sticky moment	Area for improvement, development or change	Class: KC/KNC/S/A/PO
3 May 2005	39	M	History of peptic ulcer, requests triple therapy – which one?	Best 'triple' therapy'. Test for H. pylori? Gastroscopy	KC
6 May 2005	22	M	Urethral discharge? Refer to GU clinic – how?	Referral criteria and opening times for GU clinic	KNC
18 May 2005	63	F	Persistent tennis elbow. How to inject? When?	Elbow injections	S
26 May 2005	32	M	Became impatient with him, anxiety about job/ redundancy	Don't like men being anxious – want him to pull his socks up!	A
2 June 2005	78	F	Consultation went badly – patient waiting more than half an hour in waiting room	Appointment system	PO

DISCOVERY PAGE – STICKY MOMENTS

Key:

Knowledge clinical	KC
Knowledge non-clinical	KNC
Skills	S
Attitude	A
Practice organisation	PO

Date	Patient		The sticky moment	Area for improvement, development or change	Class: KC/KNC/S/A/PO
	Age	Sex			

IDENTIFICATION OF EDUCATIONAL NEEDS

What did I identify as an educational need?	How am I going to meet this need?	What have I learned?	Have I collected the evidence of my learning in my portfolio?	Date completed
Triple therapy for peptic ulcers. Which is best?	Medline/library search Recent review article	Evidence is mixed (efficacy is dependent on sample used)	Yes	June 05
GU Unit details not available in surgery	Secretary to obtain from clinic	Importance of giving advance notice of request to unit in writing	n/a	n/a
Tennis elbow injection technique	Attend joint injection workshop	Value of advising patient of efficacy prior to injection	Yes	July 05
Anxious young man/impatient doctor	Recognise problem of attitude to this kind of patient. Discuss with partner/mentor. Communication workshop	Importance of staying calm! Importance of two way communication, using positive feedback techniques	Yes	Aug 05
Patient waiting too long in waiting room	Discuss at practice meeting. Audit waiting times and consultation interviews	Importance of early and regular audits. The value of practice meetings for practical problem solving	Yes	Sep 05

IDENTIFICATION OF EDUCATIONAL NEEDS

What did I identify as an educational need?	How am I going to meet this need?	What have I learned?	Have I collected the evidence of my learning in my portfolio?	Date completed

Blind spots

You may identify other 'needs' by using this simple checklist of blind spots, although this list is by no means exhaustive!

1 Personal skills
   - Communication, e.g. effective and appropriate telephone advice
   - Time management
   - Coping with pressure
   - Challenging patients
   - Finance
   - Personal organisation
   - Staff management
   - Navigating the NHS.

2 Clinical skills
   - Cardiopulmonary resuscitation and other basic clinical skills, e.g. fundoscopy
   - Medical knowledge.

3 New developments in primary care
   - PCOs
   - nGMS
   - Clinical governance
   - Clinical effectiveness
   - Clinical audit
   - Medicines management
   - Practice-based commissioning
   - Research and development
   - QOF points.

4 Local and national priorities
   - LDPs
   - HNAs
   - NSFs
     - Mental Health
     - Diabetes – Standards
     - Coronary Heart Disease
     - National Cancer Plan
     - Older People
     - Renal Services
     - Long-Term Conditions
     - Children.

Other methods of identifying needs are discussed in more detail further in this chapter. You may also identify needs from reading, attending journal clubs, or browsing the Internet.

Phased evaluation plan (PEP)

The Royal College of General Practitioners (RCGP) developed 'PEP', a set of educational self-assessment programmes for general practice in 1987, principally as a formative assessment tool for GP registrars. It is available to any GP who wishes to make use of it. PEP has proved to be popular and effective as a teaching instrument since its inception with both GPs and those training for general practice. It is widely used by course organisers and GP trainers both in the UK and abroad and in the armed forces. Since that time, there have been many changes in the methods of assessment within the programme.

Phased Evaluation Programme – Question Bank (PEP-QB)

PEP-QB is the latest addition (2002) to the already successful PEP range. Like PEP-2000, it will be of use to all who are working in, or preparing for a career in, general practice.

PEP-QB, available on CD-ROM, offers 160 multiple-choice questions covering the full range of clinical areas in general practice:

- Therapeutics and prescribing
- Asthma
- Practice management
- General medicine
- Dermatology
- Obstetrics and gynaecology
- Ophthalmology
- Emergency medicine
- Family planning
- Geriatric medicine
- Psychiatry
- Paediatrics
- ENT

It provides interactive self-assessment exercises with instant detailed feedback, including correct answers and recommended references for further reading.

This programme will allow you to:

- evaluate your skill level to inform your own PDP;
- use a comparative scoring system to calculate your own actual scores against your own confidence ratings; and
- work at a time of your choosing and at your own pace.

This product has been extensively tested and statistically validated to ensure your results will provide good evidence, which will help you design your own PDP.

To order a CD, contact:
RCGP Scotland
25 Queen Street
Edinburgh
EH2 1JX
Tel: 0131 260 6800
Fax: 0131 260 6836
Scottishc@rcgp.org.uk

Communication skills

A medical degree is no substitute for clairvoyance.
(George Bernard Shaw)

If you want a guarantee, buy a toaster.
(A rude doctor)

Communication is the final common pathway of everything we do and as society changes, so does our consultation behaviour. In 1871, the American physician Oliver Wendell Holmes told his students 'Your patient has no more right to all the truth you know than he has to all the medicine in your saddlebags . . . He should get only so much as is good for him'. As recently as 1993, 60% of European gastroenterologists would not routinely tell a patient he/she had cancer (Thomsen *et al.* 1993), but the only patients protected from their diagnosis today are those with dementia (Vassilas & Donaldson 1998). The agenda has moved from "What have I got?" to 'Will it work?' and even 'Are you any good at it, doctor?'

The law too is changing as the United Kingdom merges with Europe. Out will go the Bolam principle, whereby patients are told what a reasonable doctor considers is right. Instead, patients will have a right to know 'what a reason-able patient would want to know', and who would not want to know if the surgeon you are referring them to is a specialist, with figures to prove it, or a 'once-a-year bodger'? There is good evidence that "high volume" specialist surgical teams get better results than there occasional counterparts (Kileen *et al.* 2005) and if patient choice is to mean anything, it must be supported by robust and user-friendly evidence of outcomes.

So, how can you keep your communication skills up to scratch? The key unit of accountability for GPs is the primary care team, and you have to make space for honest, open discussion. Most of the communication problems encountered are not because of difficult patients, but rather difficulties between partners. As a team, you are collectively responsible for the competence of every member, and the days when you could bury or ignore worries about a colleague have gone. Poor communication in a previously happy doctor is often the first sign of stress, depression or addiction. Act before it reaches crisis point.

As for doctor–patient communication, there are several options, each of which requires a fair amount of bravery. In an ideal world, we should scrutinise each other's consultation with the same rigour we scrutinise our prescribing but many of us feel threatened by being directly observed at work. Many practices now have the technology to allow staff (not just the GPs) to video their consultations (with consent) but the key to successful analysis requires constructive feedback, a skill which a few of us are not able to manage intuitively.

However, within your primary care team, there are sure to be experienced teachers who could lend their expertise, and your local course organiser, GP tutor or university may offer the resource of simulated patients. These are usually professional actors who are trained not just to assimilate realistically a wide range of patient roles but to give constructive and insightful feedback. They can often be hired out (e.g. for an away day in a congenial setting) and used to reinvent scenarios tailored to individual members of staff. Reflect on what areas you find most difficult, and write the scenario and then do it until you feel competent. If it is done well, it can be about the best training there is.

But what about a model of analysis? All of us like the safety blanket of structure, although rarely need to resort to the harness of Pendelton's rules. Brilliant communicators are often 'unconsciously competent' but to reflect on what we are doing and share skills with others we need to be able to articulate what went on. Perhaps the following model may help:

1   Agenda (what were you trying to achieve?).
2   Outcome (what did you think you achieved?).
3   Process (which skills and tactics worked? which didn't? why not? what else might you have done?).
4   Issues (implications for you as a doctor, the team, how you cope with the job, etc.).

Context is the key to understanding communication and the twin pressures of informed consent and protocol-driven medicine are eroding holism. A GP recently sent me an anonymised letter from a neurosurgeon, with patient consent for publication:

I offered this lady an L4/5 discectomy. I have told her that the risks include, but are not limited to, complications of anaesthesia, bleeding, infection, development of any neurological deficit for example weakness and numbness of the legs, problems with the bladder or bowels, CSF leak, no improvement in current signs and symptoms, worsening of present signs and symptoms, death and other seen and unforeseen complications. She understands and wishes to proceed.

Back in primary care, the model of population-based disease management has been implemented in the new contract, and communication is in danger of being driven by the need to accrue quality points, rather than the needs of the patient. The largest ever survey of NHS patients (Picker Institute 2005) found that although trust in NHS staff is high, the manner of consultation is often still quite controlling and paternalistic, with patients desiring better information and more involvement in decision making. And all in under 10 minutes!

A final thought: observation of hundreds of students and doctors communicating has shown that the really good ones nearly always have two things in common – a life outside medicine and an ability to draw a clear distinction between work and leisure. Workaholism may be the respectable addiction, but it is as damaging as any other, so remember, no one ever said on their deathbed that they wished they had spent more time at the office.

- Do you need to take time out to brush up on your consultation skills?
- If so, why not add it to your PDP?

Medical ethics

Being a good GP is an odd compound of broad knowledge, multiple skills, deep stickability and a touch of showbiz, but even just to get by we need some understanding of how to make moral judgements. Most dramatically, we need this when there are *conflicts*: a patient makes a difficult demand, partners fall out, or the PCO board faces a choice between two vital services. Most obviously, we need such a skill when faced with *identified dilemmas*: requests for termination of pregnancy or euthanasia, the temptation to lie to a dying patient, an encounter with an uncontrolled epileptic patient who insists on driving.

Most commonly, we have *feelings of discomfort*, which alert us to something which is not right in what we are hearing or doing. But in reality almost every choice in health care, at any level, has a moral element if we look into it. A decision made carefully, with options and their logic examined and different players' perspectives taken into account, will be a better decision, while one that is slipshod, imposed, or with arguments and views only partially understood is bound to be flawed, and may come unstuck.

In addition to scientific evidence, relevant audit and appropriate clinical skills, we need to be able to detect the moral elements of a problem and weigh them carefully with the other aspects. Call it clinical governance, survival or lifelong learning, it is certainly what good practice is about.

153

Example

One of your longest serving staff has a new boyfriend who is on the practice list. Late one evening, you leave her to lock up, but return to collect something you have left behind and surprise her reading his notes. Confused and distressed, she discloses that he has been open to her about his previous bisexual lifestyle, but has been evasive when she asked about his previous partners. Someone has just told her that 'someone he was close to had died of AIDS' and she has not been able to sleep or work properly thinking about it. Unfortunately, she just has her finger on an unguarded and uncomplimentary note made in the records by the new partner.

- What sort of problems trip you up?
- What sort of issues do you have strong views about?
- Would you like to spend some time thinking about these, from different points of view (including those at variance with your own)?
- Would you like to include these in your PDP?

Resuscitation

Every GP will find that they have to manage patients with acute MI, and occasionally they may have to cope with cardiac arrest. As the latter almost always occurs unexpectedly, would you be able to cope?

The most common cause of cardiac arrest in adults is related to ischaemic heart disease, or potentially fatal rhythm abnormalities such as ventricular fibrillation or pulseless ventricular tachycardia (sudden cardiac death). Other important causes are trauma, asphyxia, choking, drug overdose, hypothermia, immersion and anaphylaxis. Respiratory causes are more common in children.

Properly managed, survival rates from out-of-hospital cardiac arrest can be of the order of 15–30%.

The key elements for survival (ABCD)

- **Immediate call for help (telephone 999 or 112).**
- **Immediate bystander basic life support to buy time.**
  Artificial ventilation using mouth to mouth (possibly with a protective shield) with a clear airway using head tilt, chin lift and jaw thrust.
  External chest compressions.
- **Early defibrillation**
  Almost all of the survivors come from those with ventricular fibrillation or pulseless ventricular tachycardia.
  Defibrillation performed very early has a high prospect of success, but survival rates fall by 7% for every minute of delay.
  Defibrillators are now automated, very simple to use and considerably cheaper than they were.
  There are many reports of the use of defibrillators by GPs with even higher success rates than the ambulance service. In addition to the ambulance service, several police forces, some fire services, airlines, airports, rail stations, shopping malls, sports centres and elements of the St John Ambulance, St Andrew's Association and the Red Cross and members of Community 'Heart Watch' schemes have now been trained and supplied with automated defibrillators.
- **Airway and ventilation with devices and oxygen**
  This is essential to prevent hypoxic damage to vital organs if the period of cardiac arrest extends for longer than about 4 minutes.
  A laryngeal mask is easy to use and is effective with a self-inflating bag valve.
- **Drug therapy**
  Drugs such as adrenaline and lidocaine have little proven value during cardiac arrest, but adrenaline is vital in severe anaphylaxis.

Are you prepared?

There is no more frightening experience for any GP than to be confronted with a patient with cardiac arrest. Make sure that you are trained in resuscitation – it will take less than 2 hours. Invest in the correct equipment.

If not, why not?

If you have not answered 'No' to most of the questions below, ask yourself if your performance would measure up to standards of best practice.

1 Are you and your staff prepared to respond to such a situation?	❏ Yes/No ❏
2 When did you last attend a course on resuscitation, or even read about what to do?	❏ Yes/No ❏
3 Have you arranged for your nurses and your reception staff to attend a course?	❏ Yes/No ❏
4 Have you acquired posters or leaflets showing what to do in a cardiorespiratory arrest?	❏ Yes/No ❏
5 Do you know how to operate an ECG defibrillator?	❏ Yes/No ❏
6 Does your practice have an ECG defibrillator?	❏ Yes/No ❏
7 Is it not time you acquired one for the emergency doctor?	❏ Yes/No ❏
8 Do you have oxygen on the premises?	❏ Yes/No ❏
9 Does the emergency duty doctor carry oxygen?	❏ Yes/No ❏
10 Do you or your nurses carry adrenaline for anaphylaxis?	❏ Yes/No ❏
11 Have you arranged for relatives of at-risk patients to be trained in basic life support?	❏ Yes/No ❏

⬣ ? Do you want to add this to your PDP?

For more information on training opportunities for you and your staff and for information about posters, leaflets and equipment, contact the resuscitation officer at your local hospital.

Conflict in the consultation – data entry vs caring

This is one of the major dilemmas facing modern professional general practice: how to care and how to record at the same time and to be effective at both?

There is a conflict between two major developments in primary care: the embracing, rigorous but formulaic evidence-based medicine and the consumerist personal autonomy-based patient-centred medicine. They can appear mutually exclusive but to be effective primary care doctors we must learn to fuse these apparently opposing views.

How to record effectively and still care

These two activities are separate behaviours and until you are skilled at amalgamation they should be treated as such. This means that the primary care consultation needs space and time for both.

The cycle of care

Modified from Pendleton DA, Schofield TPC, Tate PHL, Havelock PB (2003) *The New Consultation: Developing Doctor–Patient Communication.* The Open University Press.

Caring is about discovering what matters to your patients in a psychosocial sense and dealing effectively with these issues both medically and personally. It is about your patient's agenda. Most but not all data entry relates to the doctor's (sometimes externally imposed, e.g. contractual) agenda. The way to resolve the conflict is to manage both agendas separately and then bring them together. A brief study of the diagram above illustrates the separate agendas.

An effective consultation is one that achieves the desired outcomes for both parties. As recording will be a feature of your agenda it makes sense to make it a feature of the patient's agenda too.

Problem-orientated patient records

These were developed in the 1970s and now incorporated into several computer systems. This is a useful methodology for this sort of recording. The acronym is known as **SOAP**:

Subjective	The patient's view
Objective	The medical collection of data
Assessment	The medical synthesis, ideally with patient input
Plan	The shared outcome

The initial time of any consultation must belong to the patient, even in the disease-based clinic setting. This is the time for the patient to lay out his/her agenda and for you to listen and record what it is that matters to him/her.

The process of recording a simple precis (subjective) acts as a clarification of the patient's perceived needs and introduces the concept of sharing into the interaction.

Consulting room layout

This is important – how important research has not entirely clarified, but it seems axiomatic that if both doctors and patients want a sharing then the structure and the ambience must facilitate that.

Both parties should be able to see the screen, but there is a caveat even here: in consultations where a third party is present there is a real confidentiality issue. This means that the computer screen must be mobile and in third-party consultations explicit permission must be sought to display personal information visible to that party. Sharing information using a computer screen is a powerful tool, tends to improve recall and certainly improves evidence-based patient choice.

Doctors and patients make sense of their experiences of health and health care by developing their understanding. This forms the primary link between consultations. If there is to be less continuity of care, the onus must be on the better recording of information to allow the doctor's understanding to develop.

Recording of information

Our computers must be structured to allow the following information to be recorded.

1 What really mattered to the patient?	Subjective
2 What were their significant health beliefs?	Subjective
3 Relevant social and psychological information.	Objective
4 Appropriate clinical information.	Objective
5 Working diagnosis READ coded.	Assessment
6 Appropriate guidelines.	Plan
7 Did I use what they thought when I started explaining?	Plan
8 Did I give them the opportunity to be involved in decisions?	Plan
9 Did I explore their understanding of the diagnosis?	Plan
10 Did I explore their understanding of the treatment?	Plan
11 Did I make some attempt to see that they really understood?	Plan
12 What did we agree?	Plan

The tasks
- Understand the problem.
- Understand the patient.
- Share understanding.
- Share decisions and responsibility.
- Record the information effectively, both clinical and interpersonal.
- Maintain the relationship.
- Do all these things in an acceptable time frame.

The practice must be moving towards presenting its patients with a printout of the consultation to enhance their involvement and understanding.

The learning and teaching

This whole immensely skilful activity requires lots of practice and structured feedback to perfect. When we can achieve these tasks regularly in an acceptable time frame, then that means we have moved from being novice to expert (page 83). This transition is not magical but will require a lot of effort on both the learner's and the teacher's behalf.

Several structured consultation aids such as mapping, detailed video dissections, and patient satisfaction questionnaires can enhance and inform this learning process.

Stress and you

As a practicing health professional you will already know an awful lot about the symptoms and signs of stress. You will recognise stress in others, and to some extent in yourself. What you really need are skills to control sources of stress at work, for you and others, and to minimise its effects on you and your colleagues. More than that you need to develop the right attitude. Do not tolerate too much stress, you do not need to put up with it. It is not a fixed component of your working life in general practice.

Whether stress is altogether a bad thing depends on how much stress you are under, for how long it is applied, whether you feel powerless to stand up to the stress or can overcome it. With a modest amount of stress you are likely to perform well at work and to maintain a zest for life. No stress can be boring, whereas too much stress over too long a time will eventually render you indecisive, exhausted or burnt out.

A quick check on your symptoms of stress

The list below describes behavioural and personal symptoms of stress that some people experience. Tick the ones that you have experienced in the last year or so.

Behavioural symptoms	Personal symptoms
• Try to avoid paperwork	• Anxious
• Put things off	• Palpitations
• Indecisive	• Feel burdened
• Shunt work away	• Insomnia
• Under-perform	• Panic/hyperventilate
• Less efficient	• Less appetite
• Late for work	• Tired/drained
• Work longer but less done	• Jumpy or irritable
• Breakdown in relationships	• Difficulty concentrating
• Argumentative	• Depressed
• Accident prone	• Lost interest in sex
• Overeat	• Nausea/indigestion
• Withdraw from relationships	• Cynical
	• Lost confidence
	• Lack self-esteem
	• Feelings of helplessness

Take your list home and show to your partner or friend to see if they share your perspective. You may get more insight about symptoms and signs of stress you are experiencing by discussing this with them.

Reflect on sources of stress for you at work

Stress occurs in situations where workload is high, your control over workload is limited, and there is too little support available. An event or task like dealing with a patient complaint may create occasional high levels of stress whereas inappropriate requests for home visits may be a frequent cause of minor stress. A steady drip of stress-provoking circumstances may be just as likely to give you symptoms of stress as a crisis event.

The sort of things that health professionals commonly describe as causing them to feel stressed from work are:

- overload of work on an everyday basis;
- imposed targets from the government;
- pressure from patients' expectations;
- complex problems such as patients who misuse drugs or alcohol;
- patient complaint;
- interruptions when consulting or doing other focused work;
- mounds of practice paperwork;
- tensions between demands of career and family life, or time conflict between day job and social life;
- dealing with death and dying and other distressing conditions;
- relationship problems with colleagues;
- fear of, or actually making, mistakes; and
- fear of, or actually going through, litigation.

Can you recognise sources of stress from work?

Run your eyes down the aforementioned list and check if any or all of these are sources of stress for you. If you are unsure, ask your colleagues at work which sources they think induce stress in you or in them as a team. But check that the way they perceive stress matches your view and they are not misinterpreting stress when they really mean *being very busy* or *working in difficult circumstances.*

Why not dwell on one or two of these sources of stress that seem to apply to you? Think out or discuss with a colleague, what the current state is. Ponder on what factors bring it about or are contributing to it. What are the outcomes of that stress for you, how the team works, how patient care is delivered? What can you do to prevent, remove or minimise that source of stress from occurring? Then do something about it yourself and as a team. Great, you have just completed a significant-event audit and are well on your way to tackling stress at work!

Recognising effects of stress at work

Photocopy the following form for monitoring stress at work. Fill one in throughout each day and record any significant sources of stress and the effects at work. For example, too few appointments available first thing in the morning may lead to more home visits, more aggravation from patients or staff moaning about the appointments system – all creating stress. After several days look for any common themes or trends. Encourage other colleagues to keep similar logs. Then discuss your records as a team and discuss the negative effects of stress on the effectiveness of your work, the service, your job satisfaction and morale.

The sort of outcomes from the effects of stress at work are generally reduced productivity, lack of creativity, increased errors, poor decision-making, job dissatisfaction, poor timekeeping, disloyalty, increased sick

DAILY STRESS LOG AT WORK

Day:	Date:

Source of stress at work	Effects of stress
Comments:	

leave, more complaints, premature retirement, accidents, thefts, and organisational breakdown – such as partnership splits.

Taking control of stress

The first step in controlling stress is about becoming more aware when symptoms of stress occur, its effects, and consequent outcomes for yourself. Essentially controlling stress at work is about limiting your workload and expectations of you to sensible levels, taking more control over what you do and/or accepting others' support or help.

Some of the stress management techniques you will want to incorporate into your life are:

- Learn to relax so that you make the most of any free time.
- Stop being a perfectionist and accept being 'good enough'.
- Find time for personal and professional development. Regain your enthusiasm by learning a new skill or role. Increasing your job or personal satisfaction will help to protect you against stress.
- Look after your health. If you are unwell seek help early on.
- Reduce your work commitments – review how you spend your time outside work too.
- Be prepared to ask for help.
- Build strong mutually supportive networks at work with other colleagues.
- Communication, communication, communication.
- Learn to say 'no'. Learn to be assertive and practise often.
- Learn to delegate as much as possible.

Delegation is a difficult task to do well. Work through the following list to see how you fare.

DELEGATION SKILLS CHECKLIST

		Usually	Sometimes	Occasionally	Behavioural symptoms	Personal symptoms
1	I'm too busy to find the time to show someone else how to do it.	❑	❑	❑	❑	❑
2	I don't trust anyone else to do it as well as I can.	❑	❑	❑	❑	❑
3	I don't know what the capabilities of other people are but I have to give the tasks to them anyway.	❑	❑	❑	❑	❑
4	I want to keep control over what is happening so I have to be involved all the time.	❑	❑	❑	❑	❑
5	When I ask people to do things they keep coming back to ask me questions about how much responsibility they can take, or what they should do next.	❑	❑	❑	❑	❑
6	When I ask people to do things, they say that they are too busy, or they don't do the tasks quickly enough, so I end up doing them myself.	❑	❑	❑	❑	❑
7	I have so many out-of-work responsibilities that I feel too stressed to do my work properly.	❑	❑	❑	❑	❑

If you answered *usually* or *sometimes* to most of these questions, you need to gain further skills in delegation.

 Would you like to add the above to your PPDP?

And finally

Stress creeps up on you. You can be unaware that you are suffering the symptoms and signs described here. So think what you can do to prevent stress at work from occurring in the first place or to minimise it. Then enjoy your work.

Looking after yourself

There is no doubt that any type of stress or distraction can significantly affect the performance of health care professionals to varying degrees. It is your ultimate performance that counts!

It is important to understand the difference between performance and competence.

The difference between one's competence and performance is commonly a function of a distractor, i.e. those things that interfere with ideal function.

Competence	What one is capable of doing during an ideal patient consultation on an ideal day
Performance	What one actually does
Performance = Competence – Distractor	

Each of us has a variety of coping mechanisms to deal with our individual distractions. These coping mechanisms may vary from time to time. When coping mechanisms are inadequate or overwhelmed the result is distress, impaired performance or both.

What really counts is performance, not competence. The following questionnaires are examples of a tool that may help you identify areas of distraction or competence. Once a person is aware of a problem there may be an opportunity to change. Change often requires a shift in attitude. The ultimate goal is to have health care professionals who are happy, healthy and performing well.

Try and identify your priorities both personally and professionally. Take a few minutes to complete the following questionnaire. It is designed to increase awareness of the types of distractors that can interfere with performance and also some of the common coping mechanisms. There is no right or wrong answer or rating scale. Consider each item and become more aware. Perhaps take a risk and share your responses with a trusted colleague. Just discussing some of these issues can make a difference!

After completing the following questionnaires, have you learned anything about your performance that you may wish to add to your practice's PPDP or PDP?

MANAGING PERFORMANCE DISTRACTORS SELF-EVALUATION

Reproduced with permission from the College of Physicians and Surgeons of British Colombia and the co-authors Dr Maureen Piercey and Dr Victor Waymouth (1998).

Key:

1	Strongly disagree
2	Disagree
3	Neutral
4	Agree
5	Strongly agree
6	Unable to assess

	1	2	3	4	5	6
1 I enjoy practice as much now as I ever have	❏	❏	❏	❏	❏	❏
2 I can get locums for my practice for holiday and education time	❏	❏	❏	❏	❏	❏
3 I am satisfied with the total number of hours that I work	❏	❏	❏	❏	❏	❏
4 I have learned to cope with the 'system' that keeps placing demands on me	❏	❏	❏	❏	❏	❏
5 I am satisfied with the medical care I provide	❏	❏	❏	❏	❏	❏
6 I am not fearful of being sued or having a complaint about me	❏	❏	❏	❏	❏	❏
7 I recognise my limitations and refer patients when I am unsure	❏	❏	❏	❏	❏	❏
8 I communicate effectively with patients, their families and other health professionals	❏	❏	❏	❏	❏	❏
9 I show compassion for patients and their families	❏	❏	❏	❏	❏	❏
10 I produce medical records that are legible and that have enough information to allow a peer to understand my reasoning process for each patient encounter	❏	❏	❏	❏	❏	❏
11 All those working in my surgery understand and respect patient confidentiality	❏	❏	❏	❏	❏	❏
12 I am financially secure	❏	❏	❏	❏	❏	❏
13 I can afford to take off as much time as I need	❏	❏	❏	❏	❏	❏
14 I have a plan that will allow me to retire at a selected time	❏	❏	❏	❏	❏	❏

	1	2	3	4	5	6
15 I have no illness that interferes with the quality of my work	❏	❏	❏	❏	❏	❏
16 I have a GP who is not myself	❏	❏	❏	❏	❏	❏
17 I exercise at least 3 times per week	❏	❏	❏	❏	❏	❏
18 I seldom feel angry or irritable	❏	❏	❏	❏	❏	❏
19 I manage personal stress effectively	❏	❏	❏	❏	❏	❏
20 I do not use alcohol or drugs to deal with stress on 'bad days'	❏	❏	❏	❏	❏	❏
21 I am tolerant of other people and events most of the time	❏	❏	❏	❏	❏	❏
22 I have a colleague to discuss my problems or concerns with	❏	❏	❏	❏	❏	❏
23 I have a personal relationship that is supportive	❏	❏	❏	❏	❏	❏
24 I have interests outside of medicine that I enjoy	❏	❏	❏	❏	❏	❏
25 I am still learning, growing, gaining new perspectives and not feeling stagnant	❏	❏	❏	❏	❏	❏
26 I recognise the difference between the things I cannot control or change and those things I can influence	❏	❏	❏	❏	❏	❏
27 Reflecting on my career, I feel satisfied that my contribution has 'made a difference' and that there is purpose and meaning to my life	❏	❏	❏	❏	❏	❏
28 I set aside time on a regular basis to grow emotionally and spiritually	❏	❏	❏	❏	❏	❏
29 I am content with my life at this time	❏	❏	❏	❏	❏	❏

The following questionnaire seeks to measure your confidence in dealing with medical conditions

THE WORK OF GENERAL PRACTICE – QUESTIONNAIRE

Key:

1	I feel very confident about this
2	I feel quite confident about this
3	I need to learn a bit more about this
4	I need to learn a lot more about this

Questionnaire to measure your confidence in dealing with the following conditions

	1	2	3	4
Infectious diseases				
Childhood infections	❑	❑	❑	❑
Influenza	❑	❑	❑	❑
Gastroenteritis	❑	❑	❑	❑
Pyrexia of unknown origin glandular fever	❑	❑	❑	❑
Hepatitis A	❑	❑	❑	❑
Hepatitis B	❑	❑	❑	❑
Hepatitis C	❑	❑	❑	❑
HIV	❑	❑	❑	❑
Tropical disease	❑	❑	❑	❑
Travel jabs	❑	❑	❑	❑
Notifiable disease	❑	❑	❑	❑
'Free from Infection' certificate	❑	❑	❑	❑
Evidence-based use of antibiotics	❑	❑	❑	❑
Ear, nose and throat				
Facial pain	❑	❑	❑	❑
Catarrhal child	❑	❑	❑	❑
Otitis media	❑	❑	❑	❑
Glue ear	❑	❑	❑	❑
Tonsillitis/sore throat	❑	❑	❑	❑
Sinusitis	❑	❑	❑	❑
Deafness	❑	❑	❑	❑
Audiology/hearing aids	❑	❑	❑	❑
Hoarseness	❑	❑	❑	❑
Meniere's disease	❑	❑	❑	❑
Vertigo	❑	❑	❑	❑
Tinnitus	❑	❑	❑	❑
Hay fever	❑	❑	❑	❑
Indications for T&A	❑	❑	❑	❑
Dysphagia	❑	❑	❑	❑
Epistaxis	❑	❑	❑	❑
Eyes				
Conjunctivitis	❑	❑	❑	❑
Painful red eye	❑	❑	❑	❑
Corneal ulcers	❑	❑	❑	❑
Cataract	❑	❑	❑	❑
Squint/orthoptics	❑	❑	❑	❑

	1	2	3	4
Glaucoma	❏	❏	❏	❏
Fundoscopy	❏	❏	❏	❏
Services for partial sight	❏	❏	❏	❏
Sudden loss of vision	❏	❏	❏	❏
Floaters	❏	❏	❏	❏

Chest and breast diseases

	1	2	3	4
Acute asthma	❏	❏	❏	❏
Chronic asthma	❏	❏	❏	❏
COPD	❏	❏	❏	❏
Occupational lung diseases	❏	❏	❏	❏
TB	❏	❏	❏	❏
Bronchitis/pneumonia	❏	❏	❏	❏
Ca lung	❏	❏	❏	❏
Cough	❏	❏	❏	❏
Acute breathlessness	❏	❏	❏	❏
Screening for Ca breast	❏	❏	❏	❏
Chest pain (excl. cardiovascular)	❏	❏	❏	❏

Heart and circulation

	1	2	3	4
Hypertension	❏	❏	❏	❏
Lipids	❏	❏	❏	❏
Heart failure	❏	❏	❏	❏
Acute MI	❏	❏	❏	❏
Angina	❏	❏	❏	❏
CPR	❏	❏	❏	❏
Post-MI rehabilitation	❏	❏	❏	❏
ECGs	❏	❏	❏	❏
Peripheral vascular disease	❏	❏	❏	❏
Varicose veins	❏	❏	❏	❏
Deep vein thrombosis	❏	❏	❏	❏
Collapse	❏	❏	❏	❏
Primary prevention of heart disease	❏	❏	❏	❏
Secondary prevention of heart disease	❏	❏	❏	❏

Gynaecology/genitourinary

	1	2	3	4
Menopause/HRT	❏	❏	❏	❏
Cervical screening	❏	❏	❏	❏
Breast screening	❏	❏	❏	❏
Post-menopausal bleeding	❏	❏	❏	❏
Vaginal discharge	❏	❏	❏	❏
Dyspareunia	❏	❏	❏	❏
Impotence	❏	❏	❏	❏
Subfertility	❏	❏	❏	❏
Psychosexual problems	❏	❏	❏	❏
RELATE	❏	❏	❏	❏
Cystitis	❏	❏	❏	❏
Nephritis/pyelitis	❏	❏	❏	❏
Renal colic	❏	❏	❏	❏
Haematuria	❏	❏	❏	❏
Uterine/ovarian cancer	❏	❏	❏	❏
Bladder/prostatic cancer	❏	❏	❏	❏
Prostatism/retention	❏	❏	❏	❏
Incontinent males	❏	❏	❏	❏

	1	2	3	4
Incontinent females	❑	❑	❑	❑
Family planning				
Oral contraception	❑	❑	❑	❑
Other hormonal methods	❑	❑	❑	❑
Caps	❑	❑	❑	❑
IUCD	❑	❑	❑	❑
Sterilization	❑	❑	❑	❑
Other contraceptive methods	❑	❑	❑	❑
Under 16s	❑	❑	❑	❑
Religious/ethnic differences	❑	❑	❑	❑
Unplanned pregnancy and TOP	❑	❑	❑	❑
Obstetrics				
Antenatal care in practice	❑	❑	❑	❑
Postnatal care in practice	❑	❑	❑	❑
Home deliveries	❑	❑	❑	❑
Administration (forms/benefits/claims)	❑	❑	❑	❑
Paediatrics				
Child health surveillance	❑	❑	❑	❑
Common minor problems	❑	❑	❑	❑
Minor orthopaedic problems	❑	❑	❑	❑
Common acute emergencies	❑	❑	❑	❑
Rare but important emergencies	❑	❑	❑	❑
GP role in rare disease	❑	❑	❑	❑
Behavioural problems (sources of help)	❑	❑	❑	❑
Children Act (physical/sexual abuse)	❑	❑	❑	❑
Child protection/courts	❑	❑	❑	❑
Adoption/fostering/residential homes	❑	❑	❑	❑
The elderly				
Over-75 health surveillance	❑	❑	❑	❑
Falls in the elderly	❑	❑	❑	❑
Dementia	❑	❑	❑	❑
Elderly in own homes residential/nursing homes	❑	❑	❑	❑
Home carers	❑	❑	❑	❑
Meals on Wheels	❑	❑	❑	❑
Voluntary services and private sector	❑	❑	❑	❑
Cancer				
Early recognition/screening	❑	❑	❑	❑
Symptom relief/palliative care	❑	❑	❑	❑
GP knowledge of hospital care	❑	❑	❑	❑
Role of hospice/Macmillan nurse	❑	❑	❑	❑
Communication with patients/relatives	❑	❑	❑	❑
Abdomen				
Recurrent upper abdominal pain	❑	❑	❑	❑
Recurrent lower abdominal pain	❑	❑	❑	❑
Acute abdominal pain	❑	❑	❑	❑
Diarrhoea	❑	❑	❑	❑
Indication for investigation	❑	❑	❑	❑
Rectal bleeding	❑	❑	❑	❑
Weight loss	❑	❑	❑	❑
Central nervous system				
Epilepsy	❑	❑	❑	❑

	1	2	3	4
Hysterical fits	❑	❑	❑	❑
Headache	❑	❑	❑	❑
Migraine	❑	❑	❑	❑
Parkinson's disease	❑	❑	❑	❑
CVNTIA	❑	❑	❑	❑
Stroke rehabilitation	❑	❑	❑	❑
MS	❑	❑	❑	❑
Brain tumours	❑	❑	❑	❑
TATT	❑	❑	❑	❑

Endocrine disease

	1	2	3	4
Managing diabetes	❑	❑	❑	❑
Complication of diabetes	❑	❑	❑	❑
GP diabetic clinics	❑	❑	❑	❑
Hypothyroidism	❑	❑	❑	❑
Hyperthyroidism	❑	❑	❑	❑
Hyperprolactinaemia	❑	❑	❑	❑
Delayed puberty	❑	❑	❑	❑

Musculoskeletal

	1	2	3	4
Rheumatoid				
Osteoarthritis	❑	❑	❑	❑
Gout	❑	❑	❑	❑
Osteoporosis	❑	❑	❑	❑
Back pain	❑	❑	❑	❑
Neck/shoulder pain	❑	❑	❑	❑
Physiotherapy	❑	❑	❑	❑
Local injections	❑	❑	❑	❑
Tendon inflammation	❑	❑	❑	❑
Complementary medicine	❑	❑	❑	❑
ME/fibromyalgia	❑	❑	❑	❑
Joint injections	❑	❑	❑	❑
Periarticular injection	❑	❑	❑	❑

Diseases of the mind

	1	2	3	4
Anxiety	❑	❑	❑	❑
Depression	❑	❑	❑	❑
Insomnia	❑	❑	❑	❑
Atypical presentations of depression	❑	❑	❑	❑
Abuse of prescribed drugs	❑	❑	❑	❑
Abuse of illicit drugs	❑	❑	❑	❑
Alcohol abuse	❑	❑	❑	❑
Smoking	❑	❑	❑	❑
Eating disorders	❑	❑	❑	❑
Managing the disturbed patient	❑	❑	❑	❑
Counselling	❑	❑	❑	❑
Family therapy	❑	❑	❑	❑
Mental health team	❑	❑	❑	❑
Care in the community	❑	❑	❑	❑

Skin disease

	1	2	3	4
Acne	❑	❑	❑	❑
Eczema	❑	❑	❑	❑
Psoriasis	❑	❑	❑	❑
Warts	❑	❑	❑	❑

	1	2	3	4
Skin disease (continued)	❏	❏	❏	❏
Infestations	❏	❏	❏	❏
Fungal infections	❏	❏	❏	❏
Leg ulcers	❏	❏	❏	❏
Skin cancer	❏	❏	❏	❏
Urticaria/angioedema	❏	❏	❏	❏
Pruritus	❏	❏	❏	❏
Rosacea	❏	❏	❏	❏
Emollients	❏	❏	❏	❏
Drug rashes	❏	❏	❏	❏
In-growing toenails	❏	❏	❏	❏
Sebaceous cysts	❏	❏	❏	❏
Skin biopsy	❏	❏	❏	❏
Incision of abscess	❏	❏	❏	❏
Treating warts	❏	❏	❏	❏
Minor surgery – Organisation & equipment	❏	❏	❏	❏
Minor surgery – Competence & accreditation	❏	❏	❏	❏

Investigation

	1	2	3	4
X-ray (use and abuse)	❏	❏	❏	❏
Availability (e.g. Ba enema)	❏	❏	❏	❏
Endoscopy	❏	❏	❏	❏
Ultrasound	❏	❏	❏	❏

Therapeutics

	1	2	3	4
Practice formularies	❏	❏	❏	❏
Doctor's emergency drugs	❏	❏	❏	❏
PACT	❏	❏	❏	❏
Role of pharmacist	❏	❏	❏	❏
Product liability	❏	❏	❏	❏
Monitoring repeat prescribing	❏	❏	❏	❏
Alternatives to drugs	❏	❏	❏	❏
Generic/branded private	❏	❏	❏	❏
POM/P	❏	❏	❏	❏
General/black list	❏	❏	❏	❏
ACBS	❏	❏	❏	❏
Cost-benefit analysis	❏	❏	❏	❏
Controlled drug regulations	❏	❏	❏	❏
Prescription charges/exemptions	❏	❏	❏	❏
Personally administered items	❏	❏	❏	❏

Disability and handicap

	1	2	3	4
Medical certificates	❏	❏	❏	❏
Disability Resettlement Officer	❏	❏	❏	❏
Maternity benefit	❏	❏	❏	❏
Sickness benefits	❏	❏	❏	❏
Invalidity benefits	❏	❏	❏	❏
Disability benefits	❏	❏	❏	❏
Attendance allowance (+ special rules)	❏	❏	❏	❏
Mobility allowance/motability	❏	❏	❏	❏
Disease-oriented groups	❏	❏	❏	❏
Self-help groups	❏	❏	❏	❏
Caring for carers	❏	❏	❏	❏

	1	2	3	4
Residential homes for children/young adults	❏	❏	❏	❏
Fitness to drive	❏	❏	❏	❏
Fit to travel by air	❏	❏	❏	❏

Prevention, screening, patient education

	1	2	3	4
Criteria for a screening test	❏	❏	❏	❏
Opportunistic screening/case finding	❏	❏	❏	❏
Targets	❏	❏	❏	❏
Practice leaflet	❏	❏	❏	❏
Newsletter	❏	❏	❏	❏

Medical ethics

	1	2	3	4
Confidentiality (relatives/insurers/police etc.)	❏	❏	❏	❏
Minors (contraception)	❏	❏	❏	❏
Consent to treatment	❏	❏	❏	❏
Euthanasia	❏	❏	❏	❏
Rationing care	❏	❏	❏	❏
TOP	❏	❏	❏	❏
Ethics committee and research	❏	❏	❏	❏
Chaperones	❏	❏	❏	❏
Dispensing by GPS	❏	❏	❏	❏

Organization of the NHS

	1	2	3	4
DoH	❏	❏	❏	❏
SHA	❏	❏	❏	❏
NHS funding streams	❏	❏	❏	❏
PCO	❏	❏	❏	❏
Clinical governance	❏	❏	❏	❏
LMC	❏	❏	❏	❏
GMC	❏	❏	❏	❏
GPC	❏	❏	❏	❏
CHI	❏	❏	❏	❏
Workforce Development Federations	❏	❏	❏	❏
NICE	❏	❏	❏	❏
Community (GP) hospitals	❏	❏	❏	❏
NHSDirect	❏	❏	❏	❏
Walk-In Centres	❏	❏	❏	❏

Practice Staff

	1	2	3	4
Employing staff	❏	❏	❏	❏
Staff Appraisal	❏	❏	❏	❏
Role of practice managers	❏	❏	❏	❏
Role of practice nurses	❏	❏	❏	❏
Role of health visitors	❏	❏	❏	❏
Role of Reception Staff	❏	❏	❏	❏
Role of district nurses	❏	❏	❏	❏
Role of community midwives	❏	❏	❏	❏
Contracts of employment	❏	❏	❏	❏
Disciplinary procedures	❏	❏	❏	❏

Practice organization

	1	2	3	4
Cooperatives and providers of out of Hours	❏	❏	❏	❏
Nurse triage	❏	❏	❏	❏
Contacting doctors (bleeps, etc.)	❏	❏	❏	❏
Partnership agreement	❏	❏	❏	❏

	1	2	3	4
Appointments systems	❏	❏	❏	❏
Patients records	❏	❏	❏	❏
Registers of age/sex or morbidity	❏	❏	❏	❏
Recall systems	❏	❏	❏	❏
Medical insurances	❏	❏	❏	❏
Medicolegal reports	❏	❏	❏	❏
NSFs	❏	❏	❏	❏
HNAs	❏	❏	❏	❏
LDPs	❏	❏	❏	❏
Audit	❏	❏	❏	❏
Types of practice	❏	❏	❏	❏
Training practice	❏	❏	❏	❏
Health and safety at work	❏	❏	❏	❏
NHS funding for surgery premises	❏	❏	❏	❏
Managing time	❏	❏	❏	❏
Managing change	❏	❏	❏	❏
Managing stress	❏	❏	❏	❏
Complaints	❏	❏	❏	❏
Non-sessional doctors	❏	❏	❏	❏
COSSH	❏	❏	❏	❏

nGMS

	1	2	3	4
Read codes	❏	❏	❏	❏
Essential services	❏	❏	❏	❏
Additional services	❏	❏	❏	❏
QOF points	❏	❏	❏	❏

Accounts and taxation

	1	2	3	4
NHS pension scheme for GPs	❏	❏	❏	❏
NHS pension scheme for staff	❏	❏	❏	❏
Cash flow	❏	❏	❏	❏
MPIG payments	❏	❏	❏	❏
PPIFs	❏	❏	❏	❏

Use of computers

	1	2	3	4
Anti-virus protection	❏	❏	❏	❏
Firewalls	❏	❏	❏	❏
Password policy	❏	❏	❏	❏
Use of Internet	❏	❏	❏	❏
Practice website	❏	❏	❏	❏

Useful websites for *Methods of identifying educational needs*

Phased Evaluation Plan (PEP)	www.rcgp-scotland.org.uk/products/pep
Royal College of General Practice (RCGP)	www.rcgp.org.uk
Royal College of Nursing (RCN)	www.rcn.org.uk

A full list of websites can be found on pages 192–197.

Meeting educational and developmental needs

Many people fear that using a PDP and becoming a self-directed learner means that they will be forever consigned to a life of lonely private study, missing out on enjoyable interaction with colleagues on study days. Others fear that having identified their learning needs, they will be unable to find suitable courses to attend to fulfil them, leading to failure and increased awareness of their inadequacies. Many health professionals also fear that their learning needs are infinite and disparate; that is, each person would have wide-ranging needs which would not be shared by their colleagues. They therefore feel that it was not worthwhile to try to assess their needs and plan how to meet them, as this would be impossible. No one, least of all local GP tutors, would ever be able to run enough courses to meet all of these varied needs.

Having decided what your learning needs are, how then should you meet them? This broadly depends on five factors:

- Your learning style – how you prefer to learn.
- Your learning skills – how effective you are at directing and organising your learning.
- What the learning need is – a small specific question or a general need for updating.
- What your learning goal is – this might include some form of external certification or examination.
- What's available to you?

Learning style

It might be worthwhile spending the time completing a learning style inventory to find out what your learning style is. By identifying your learning style you may become aware that you have particular problems with getting the most of learning, however you are approaching it. Most health care professionals, because of their wide experience of learning and study, are able to adapt to many different types of learning and so although you may have a preference for lectures over discussions or reading, you are probably able to benefit from a case discussion or reading a paper. Nearly everyone benefits from learning about the same thing in different ways as this helps us to practice using new information and so reinforces the learning. This is why so many courses are organised with a mixture of lectures and interactive sessions, which may seem to cover the same ground.

Learning skills – getting the most out of your learning

Do not approach a study day or a lecture with the idea that you must retain all the detailed information presented during the session. On the other hand, do not deliberately start the session with your mind entirely empty of expectations. In order to learn and change our ideas, we need to integrate new ideas with old. As an experienced health care professional, you will very rarely be presented with a session in which all of the material is entirely new to you – you will always have some relevant knowledge.

To get the most out of a learning session – whether this is a study day, a single lecture or even some private reading – two things are needed: some preparation beforehand and some reflection afterwards.

Preparation – this should take only a few minutes. You can do this the night before, or even take a few minutes sitting in the car park at the venue. You can also do this before you read that journal article or book or start the online study module:

- Read through the information you have about the lecture or course – especially any aims and objectives.
- Recall what it was that stimulated you to think you should attend it.
- Remind yourself of the previously identified learning need you are trying to fulfil.
- Make brief notes of what *you* want to get out of the session.
- If you have time, it is useful to write down some brief notes on what you already know about the subject – '*cognitive mapping*'.

During the session, try to pay particular attention to the material that answers your needs. If you still have unanswered questions or unmet needs at the end, then ask about these during any discussion or question time. Cognitive mapping will highlight areas in your knowledge base that are lacking or out of date. It is then easier to integrate the new knowledge with the old and update your ideas.

Reflection

Once again, something taking a few minutes. At the end of the session or soon afterwards complete a 'Reflective Practice' form; the form on page 51 might be helpful.

Get out the notes you made beforehand and during the session. Keep your notes with your PDP and present it when you come to your appraisal.

Spending this time will help you to remember the new information and will make it more likely that you will be able to make changes to your practice as a result. Some study days and courses run by the more enlightened educators already include time within the day for preparation and reflection.

Your learning need

Health care professionals and in particular GPs have two types of learning needs: *general* and *specific*.

- **General** needs include things like needing an update on diabetes because you realise that patients are being given new drugs about which you know nothing and need to find out. You have a lot of questions and uncertainties about this – what are the drugs? Why should they be used? Which patients can benefit? You also have an uneasy feeling of being out of touch with up-to-date diabetes management.
- **Specific** needs usually arise in consultations with patients – perhaps a question about a possible side effect or drug interaction.

The **learning method** you undertake for these different needs will obviously vary:

- **General needs** – answered by:
  - Courses and conferences
  - Online courses
  - Distance learning courses
  - Working with an 'expert' for several sessions – e.g. sitting in on clinics
  - 'Corridor learning'
- **Specific needs** – answered by:
  - Looking it up – in a book or using online resources
  - Consulting a guideline or care pathway
  - Asking a colleague
  - Asking an 'expert'

We are very quick to address specific needs – you probably do not realise you are doing it most of the time!

Your learning goal

When you choose how to learn, you should also consider what your goal is. For example, you want to learn more about rheumatology. This could be because:

- You're not sure how to investigate Mrs Jones' painful fingers.
- You'd like to work as a clinical assistant.
- You're not sure how to assess patients with knee pain.

If it is just about Mrs Jones, you might find that some very brief reading or online courses or perhaps a chat with a more expert colleague or specialist would be enough. If your goal is to be a clinical assistant, you will probably want to consider a much more structured and long-term course, perhaps resulting in an examination and the award of a diploma. If you want to learn more about assessing patients with bad knees, then spending some time examining patients with a GP colleague, physiotherapist, rheumatologist or orthopaedic surgeon would probably be a good way to learn. A half- or one-day course would also be helpful.

Having learning goals also means knowing when to stop. You need to be realistic about what you want to achieve. You do not have to be a world expert on knee pains; you just need to know enough to cope with the everyday problems which present, and to know who to ask, where to go, for further help when necessary.

What is available to you

In the above example, you might really want to go on a one-day course about knee pains. However, nothing is available. You therefore have to work with what you have got. You might try to spend some time with someone more expert or doing some reading. You might ask around your practice and find that you are not the only one who has this need. If you have time set aside for educational meetings, perhaps you could arrange to cover knee problems at one of those meetings? Perhaps one of the local consultants and a physiotherapist would come and speak to you all together.

Conclusion

It is important to choose very carefully how you are going to spend your precious study time to get the most out of it.

- Set clear goals.
- Consider what you already know.
- Think about what you have learned.

- Do not attend courses at random because you are sure they will be interesting anyway.
- Be realistic about what you can expect to achieve.
- Try to choose a variety of different learning experiences throughout the year.
- Remember, learning should be enjoyable and to some extent relaxing.
- Try to learn 'close to home' with your practice team if possible, as it is very time efficient and can also help with team building.
  Many methods can be valuable, such as:
- Lectures
- Workshops
- Small group work
- Young principal groups
- Peer support groups
- Practice meetings
- Clinical assistantships/individual attachments
- Clinical audits
- Research
- Journal club
- Medline/Internet searches
- Using e-mail
- Distance learning courses
- Individual reading
- Appraisal
- Working in another practice
- Working with other professionals
- Diploma or masters courses

This list is by no means exhaustive and some other methods are discussed in more detail below.

Mentoring

Mentoring is defined as:

> The process whereby an experienced, highly regarded, empathic person (the mentor) guides another individual (the mentee) in the development and re-examination of their own ideas, learning, and personal and professional development. The mentor, who often but not necessarily works in the same organization or field as the mentee, achieves this by listening and talking in confidence to the mentee.

Mentoring can form a valuable part of a framework of support but should be entirely voluntary and not imposed, with confidentiality an essential part of the process. Both mentors and mentees should fully understand the purpose and limits of the mentoring relationship, and those volunteering to become mentors should be given appropriate assistance to develop their skills. Associate directors and GP tutors may be contacted for advice.

Different kinds of support are likely to be needed at different points in someone's career. Extra support may well be necessary for newly appointed GPs but can also be valuable for other members of the primary health care team.

A suitable time and place is important, and thought should be given to building appropriate amounts of time into people's work programmes. The length and frequency of mentoring meetings are likely to depend on individual needs and preferences.

Self-directed learning groups

Many health care professionals may be familiar with this style of working in preparation for examinations.

Essentially, a small group (ideally four or five) of like-minded people may wish to meet on a regular basis to share some of the workload of meeting their educational needs. This may also be particularly relevant to sessional doctors who may not regularly have the opportunity to ruminate over clinical situations in a practice setting.

The group could decide which needs may be met. Examples could be:

- researching evidence-based topics;
- therapeutics;
- journal review; and
- case discussion, e.g. clinical, ethical, etc.

It may be appropriate for each group member in turn to prepare material in advance.

Keeping up to date

This is a challenge! Reading the entire contents of this book would take you quite a time. We have to keep up to date – our peers and our patients expect us to and surely it is a matter of professional pride to be abreast of medical developments. There is no easy answer to the problem of how to do it. We need to find the time to browse the journals, but fitting it into the busy work schedule is not easy. Only you can arrange your timetable for this.

- There are innumerable journals available. The classic heavyweights such as the *British Medical Journal* and the *British Journal of General Practice* are obvious choices for the reader. However, there are a number of regular review journals that give information on current clinical practice or review articles. There are so many to choose from that personal preference is what matters.
- Gather a collection of articles that are of interest and build them into a personal reference library.
- Run a journal club on a regular basis in-house or with other practitioner groups. This generates interest and feedback can be useful.
- Get reports from colleagues who have perhaps attended a course or conference. Often we can get a distillation of new ideas and procedures, which can be very useful for all.
- Use the Internet. More and more websites are available which include access to specified journals.
- Patients will often ask about new treatments that they have seen reported in the newspapers, on TV or have read about on the Internet. This offers stimulus to find out more about these new concepts. Useful websites can be found on page 192.
- In practice, we are often faced with problems for which there is no immediate answer. These are collectively known as 'sticky moments' as described on page 144. Where there are obvious blanks, be they large or small, make a note of them for answering later.
- Your local Postgraduate Medical Education library and others offer help with searches and other references.

- How are you planning to keep up to date?
- How much time are you prepared to commit?
- How will you collect the evidence of your reading?
- Are you going to include this in your PDP?

- Representatives often have a lot of information on specific subjects and handouts can be quite informative.
- We learn and keep ahead in different ways. There is no hard and fast rule about how to do this, only to recognize the need to manage your own learning in the best way to suit you.

Higher professional education (HPE)

When first conceived, training for general practice was intended to last for 5 years, 2 in hospital posts and 3 in 'higher professional training'. Despite this, vocational training when introduced had a statutory period of 3 years. The RCGP recommended again that training for general practice should last for 5 years. The intervening years have produced a long literature demonstrating that this period is inadequate to prepare new GPs for their task. By 1995 there was wide acceptance of the need to extend the period of training for general practice. Additional work described problems of new GPs, and proposed some solutions. These included identifying and addressing needs of the 'trained' doctors. Responses to inadequate preparation have included HPE courses, vocational training scheme extensions (trainer or registrar led) and a range of 'innovative posts'.

Higher professional education courses

At least five models of higher professional education have been described:

1 An extended or enhanced period of vocational training, e.g. London's LIZEI Scheme.
2 An extended period of academic training (diplomas and higher degrees), e.g. the London Academic Training Scheme (LATS).
3 Extended personal development and assistance for failing practices, e.g. Mersey Parachute Scheme.
4 Support for new principals and sessional doctors in their first year in practice based around small group work.
5 Support for established principals and sessional doctors in their later years of practice based around small group work.

The characteristics of successful schemes have been identified through many evaluations that have examined both the new principals and the views of their senior partners. Schemes should ideally include:

- The involvement of new principals and non-career grade doctors including sessional doctors and locums.
- Protected time and adequate funding, including locum payments.
- A learner-centred agenda, with a flexible syllabus and some self-directed and some led sessions.
- The availability of flexible teaching and learning methods.
- Peer support; mentoring.
- Portfolio development.
- Liaison with other agencies.
- Appropriate quality assurance systems.

Structure of courses – the current initiative

The national HPE scheme is open to any GP during the first year after qualifying from vocational training, and provides 20 days of protected study time over that year. Service replacement costs are provided to practices at a current rate of £250 per day along with an allowance of £450 for each doctor to spend on educational materials or course fees in 2004.

Most deaneries are now running these courses, and as with the schemes that preceded this, early evaluations are strongly indicative of success.

Development

The move towards some form of extended training period has developed in response to changes in role and recognition of educational needs. These are identified by the learners and stem from the expansion of both clinical and managerial responsibilities, IT, developments in e-learning, and the requirement to address appraisal/revalidation using more formal processes than before. Evaluation of earlier courses has confirmed that relevant and appropriate topics are chosen by groups for study. These often represent attitudinal and skills-based needs within the following areas:

- Developing and writing a PDP/preparing for appraisal and revalidation.
- Management issues: personal and professional.
- GPs with a special interest (GPSIs).
- Working with and within PCOs.
- Learning and teaching skills.
- Pastoral care/support.

The near universal appreciation given to HPE schemes lends strong support for the continuation of this initiative. The following table shows where this fits into a lifelong educational programme. The availability of protected time and a realistic level of funding is vital for continued success of this scheme.

An educational time line of a medical career:

Duration	Five years	Two years	Three years	One to two years	Remainder of professional life
Situation	Medical school	Foundation years	Vocational training	Higher professional education	Continuing professional development
Position	Student	Supervised learner	Supervised/independent learner	Independent learner	Independent learner
Assessment processes	Final examinations	Undecided	Summative assessment, MRCGP	Revalidation and appraisal processes	Revalidation and appraisal processes

Career pathways
Sessional doctors

Sessional GPs (formerly known as non-principals) are an important and growing part of the GP workforce, comprising:

- assistants;
- locums;
- associate GPs;
- salaried doctors;
- GP registrars; and
- retained and flexible scheme doctors.

Wherever possible, sessional doctors should be invited to participate and contribute to team activities, such as SEA, PHCT away days and PDPs. Although sessional doctors may lose remuneration through attending these, they can gain much insight into primary care and enhance their personal portfolios and lifelong learning; the team will gain by the fresh insights sessional doctors can bring.

Sessional doctors should build on their GP registrar workbook or portfolio to develop the concept of lifelong learning, use the PDP section of this book, and attend as many team events as they can, recording these using the 'reflective practice principles'. This living, ongoing record of lifelong learning will stand them in good stead with revalidation.

Portfolio careers

Portfolio careers are a concept familiar to many GPs. A portfolio career GP frequently spends time outside the practice in activities that use a broad range of skills in different environments. Examples are occupational health work, course organization, medical politics, school health clinics and sports medicine.

A portfolio changes over time as new interests are picked up and others dropped to make space. Work patterns also change to fit in with family and other activities. Indeed, portfolio careers allow flexibility in working patterns and interests and depend on an ability to reflect on skills and strengths rather than roles. Variation in workplaces and changes in tasks maintain interest and enthusiasm.

There are downsides, as a portfolio career usually means less security. Working with different people can be fun, but it means working on more than one set of relationships.

The standard format of appraisal and job planning may not fit comfortably with a portfolio career. However, a mentor who is willing to spend time with you can be extremely effective. Considering your portfolio at regular intervals gives the opportunity to reflect on the new skills gained and how they might be used in other areas. It also gives an opportunity to consider career moves and how additions to a career portfolio will strengthen your curriculum vitae.

It is important to be honest about aspirations, and realistic about flexibility. Building up skills that could lead in more than one direction prevents focus into one career path. The same principles apply as to any other professional development.

- What do I want to achieve in the next year?
- How will it fit in with my current role in the NHS?
- What additional knowledge and skills do I want to learn?
- How will I measure success?

The difference may be that some of the new skills may be learned through working in a new area or by expanding an existing area. Two additional questions might be asked:

- Are there new opportunities coming up that I might apply for?
- What could I stop doing to make the time for the new opportunity?

General practice lends itself to portfolio careers; however, it is easy to allow them to develop without too much planning. This can be the cause of disagreements and disgruntlement in the practice and if you are contemplating building your own portfolio, consider the options available to you and how you might build towards an overall goal.

Job sharing

Job sharing is becoming more popular. Whereas part-timers would work independently of each other, job sharers operate as 'one', sharing a list of patients, appointments, office and 'vote'. To be successful this requests a common approach such as clinical styles, philosophies and probably lifestyles. A job share between two women with young children is more likely to work well than one between a junior partner with domestic commitments and a senior partner taking on more golf as he approaches retirement.

GPs with special interest (GPSIs)

GPSIs have additional training and expertise that enables them to provide and deliver a high-quality, improved access service to meet the needs of a single PCO or group of PCOs. They may deliver a clinical service beyond the normal scope of general practice, undertake advanced procedures or develop services.

They will work as partners in a managed service not under direct supervision, keeping within their competencies. They do not offer a full consultant service and will not replace consultants or interfere with access to consultants by local GPs.

If a GP has a special clinical interest that they wish to offer to PCOs, they should make themselves known to local PCOs. PCOs may wish to include information on the availability of skills in deciding how best they can develop services locally, but the appointment of a GPSI should follow a review of health needs, local service provision, and commissioning options.

GPSIs will be either employed by PCOs or acute trusts, usually on a sessional basis, or will deliver services as independent contractors. The contract that is used needs to be congruent with that of main stream hospital practitioners, in particular annual and study leave entitlement, audit, clinical governance and appraisal arrangement.

GPSIs will be principals in general practice or be eligible to be so . They must be generalists first and foremost who undertake their special interests in addition.

The following are the areas considered most likely to be priorities in terms of national programmes or services with significant access problems, although not exhaustive:

- Cardiology
- Care of the elderly
- Diabetes
- Palliative care and cancer
- Mental health (including substance misuse)
- Dermatology
- Musculoskeletal medicine
- Women and child health, including sexual health
- Ear, nose and throat
- Care for the homeless, asylum seekers, travellers and others who find access to traditional health services difficult

Other procedures suitable for a community setting are endoscopy, cystoscopy, echocardiography, vasectomy, and so on.

Teaching PCOs

At the time of writing there are some 31 teaching PCOs across the UK which are able to offer GPs and other health care professionals' clinical posts that involve teaching, research or development and represent further career development opportunities for GPs and PHCTs.

GP retainer and flexible career schemes

These schemes have produced a new group of doctors working in primary care. These part-time educational schemes help to promote flexibility, which is now needed to retain the GP workforce. Many GPs are no longer prepared to work in a profession, which traditionally embraced long hours and had a culture that could lead to stress, ill health and relationship problems. Protected time for educational activities helps to maintain a workforce that is fit for the purpose. Both schemes have an emphasis on education and supervision, with the benefit of retaining qualified GPs in the workforce. The schemes provide GPs with the opportunity to work in general practice while balancing their work and personal commitments. The deaneries are responsible for managing the schemes locally and many have appointed tutors to help monitor the schemes. There are contractual differences between the two schemes, which are beyond the remit of this book.

The GP Retainer Scheme was designed to ensure that doctors who are only able to undertake a limited amount of paid professional work could keep in touch with general practice in order to retain their skills. The retainee works in a supernumerary capacity and the scheme combines clinical and educational components. Retainees work in practices where they receive regular support and input from a named GP who acts as their educational facilitator and (or) clinical supervisor. The practice should be able to offer the retainee a full range of general medical services, including home visits where appropriate.

The Flexible Career Scheme for GPs was launched by the DoH in 2002 and provides additional supported part-time posts for GPs. The scheme was implemented in response to the recruitment and retention crisis in general practice, the improving working lives initiative as well as new national legislation relating to flexible and family friendly employment. Doctors employed on the Flexible Career Scheme work in a substantive capacity in general practice.

Approval to join the schemes

Practices can be approved to join one or both schemes if they can demonstrate that they comply with, or are working towards, the modified Joint Committee on Postgraduate Training for General Practice's (JCPTGP) minimum educational criteria for training practices. All training practices and many practices that teach undergraduates should already meet these criteria. It may be necessary for the deanery to organise a visit to other practices in order to ascertain the practice's suitability to join one or both schemes.

The deanery also determines an individual GP's eligibility to enter one of the schemes. However, doctors employed on the schemes must be eligible to work in general practice and be on the PCOs' GP performers' list.

Supervision

A named person (usually a GP) who works regularly within the practice is appointed as the educational facilitator. The deanery will need to be satisfied that the educational supervisor has the appropriate educational skills, is aware of their individual responsibilities and the aims of the schemes. A named GP within the practice is appointed as the clinical supervisor and is often, but not always, the same person as the educational supervisor. The clinical supervisor should be available for their GP retainee to provide help and advice during surgeries and at the end of the session to discuss problems and interesting cases. Flexible Career Scheme doctors may work alone in surgery, although they should still be given the opportunity to discuss issues that have arisen with their clinical supervisor at a later date.

Protected time should be made available for both the educational facilitator and the supervised doctor so that they can meet on a regular basis at a mutually convenient time for tutorials, feedback, case discussion and other aspects of general practice. The educational facilitator should help formulate a PDP designed to review the previous year's work, set learning objectives for the coming year and give the supervised doctor the opportunity to discuss their career progress and future plans. In the future the appraisal process will take on the role of formulating the PDP.

GPs on both schemes need to demonstrate that they have been involved in continuing professional development and have produced a PDP. The retainee undertakes 28 hours of education annually and Flexible Career Scheme doctors have a minimum of 8 fully funded sessions of education. Under the nGMS all salaried GPs are entitled to one session per work pro rata of protected professional development and this includes retained and Flexible Career Scheme doctors.

Funding for course fees is at the discretion of the practices, PCOs and deaneries, but in some cases the individual doctor has to bear the cost. Educational activities should be based on the doctor's PDP and may include:

- Tutorials
- Audit
- Private study
- Significant-event analysis
- Blind spots and sticky moments
- Practice educational meetings
- Preparation for appraisal
- Courses
- Career counselling
- Mentoring
- IT training
- PCO educational activities
- Sitting in with colleagues
- Clinical refresher experience
- Deanery away days
- Self-directed learning groups

The DoH will be issuing prescribing numbers to all GP performers, including retained GPs and Flexible Career Scheme doctors. All GPs will then be able to receive their own PACT data, which will be a valuable tool for appraisal and revalidation. However, owing to technical issues, the start date had not been agreed at the time of writing.

Benefits of the schemes

Offering improved working conditions with family-friendly hours in an educationally supportive practice is one of the strategies that practices and PCOs can use to attract and retain staff. The flexibility of the schemes, particularly the Flexible Career Scheme, can be used as a recruitment tool and it is hoped that the Flexible Career Scheme will enable practices to be more creative about the way they work.

Older GPs who wish to reduce their commitment and work more flexibly as they near retirement can also take the opportunity to join the FCS. These doctors have a wealth of experience and may be educators in their own right. They are often happy to work increased sessions during school holidays in return for longer holidays during term time. This can be an enormous benefit to practices that have doctors with young families.

Retained doctors can do a limited amount of non-GMS work at the discretion of the deanery's director, while doctors on the Flexible Career Scheme are allowed greater flexibility to undertake non-GMS work. In both schemes doctors can become undergraduate teachers and appraisers, which may help encourage them to become GP trainers in the future.

GP trainer

The success of the NHS is dependent on the high quality of general practice available in the UK. More GPs are needed and to supply those GPs, training capacity must be increased. High-quality training is vital if we are to produce the next generation of GPs who will be able to meet the diverse demands of primary care in the future.

Being a GP trainer is immensely rewarding, and there are benefits to the whole practice. The trainer has the pleasure of helping the GP registrar develop into a doctor who can practice independently as a GP. Having a GP registrar stimulates the trainer's own professional development. Most trainers believe that they learn as much from their registrars as the registrars learn from them. After all, it is increasingly likely that the GP registrar will bring a wealth of previous experience, both medical and non-medical to the practice. Although the GP registrar is supernumerary, and certainly during the early months will not make a significant overall contribution to the number of patients seen (particularly considering the time that the trainer will have to give to tutorials), as the year progresses and confidence grows, the GP registrar will often make an important contribution to the running of the practice.

There are other benefits that accrue to the training practice. As well as having the GP registrar's salary reimbursed, there is also a trainer's grant available to GP trainers. In addition, many training practices have found that when they need to recruit a new partner (or salaried doctor), previous GP registrars are keen to return to the practice.

In becoming a trainer, a GP has to meet certain national standards (currently laid down by the JCPTGP), which may be added to by the local deanery General Practice Education Committee. These standards involve assessing the GP as a doctor, the GP as a teacher, and the practice environment. The local deanery will be supportive in helping GPs to apply and there will be courses that the prospective trainer will need to attend. It is usual for trainers to be expected to hold the MRCGP.

For the more adventurous . . . career breaks
Sabbatical in general practice

'Taking a sabbatical in general practice' was published in the *BMJ*'s career focus in 1998. The details about prolonged study leave allowance for GPs are out of date, but it is a good place to start your planning process.

For more details regarding payments for subbatreals, contact your local PCO

Working in other countries

The 'BMJ careers' section also carries posts for GPs to work abroad.

The RCGP international committee

Provides educational exchange and dialogue between individual doctors, agencies and medical organisations in the UK and overseas. It also promotes the standing and the study of general practice/family medicine, and offers travel scholarships.

Expedition medicine

There are opportunities overseas with our range of expedition and adventure travel organisations. One contact is the ExpeList bulletin.

Relief work

Medecins Sans Frontieres is an international medical aid agency with a reputation of not only being the first to arrive in a crisis-hit area, but often, the only organisation to be there at all.

Merlin exists to provide an immediate and effective response to medical emergencies throughout the world.

Useful websites for *Meeting educational and developmental needs*

BMJ Careers	http://www.bmjcareers.com/cgi-bin/section.pl?sn=home
Expelis	www.voyageconcepts.co.uk/expeList.htm
International Health Exchange	www.ihe.org.uk
Medecins Sans Frontieres	www.doctorswithoutborders.org www.msf.org/
Merlin	www.merlin.org.uk
National Association of Sessional GPs NASGP *(formerly known as the National Association of Non Principals – NANP)*	www.nasgp.org.uk
RCGP International committee	http://www.rcgp.org.uk/international/index.asp
VSO	http://www.vso.org.uk/

A full list of websites can be found on pages 192–197.

Personal development plan

You may now wish to write your PDP by considering all the sections in this manual, which may have helped you to identify your educational and development needs.

These will form an important link to the PPDP.

	What is the key thing I have identified?	What is my goal?	How am I going to tackle this?	Target date	What will hinder me?	Action needed
Past educational profile						
Learning highlights of the past few years						
Self-audit and SCOT analysis						
Sticky moments						
Blind spots						
Phased evaluation plan						
Communication skills						
Medical ethics						
Resuscitation						
Conflict in the consultation – Data entry vs caring						
Stress and you						
Looking after yourself						

	What is the key thing I have identified?	What is my goal?	How am I going to tackle this?	Target date	What will hinder me?	Action needed
Managing performance distractors self-evaluation						
The work of general practice questionnaire						
Career pathways						

Appendix 1: Confidentiality declaration

I give permission for my Personal Development Plan to be seen for assessment and revalidation purposes by

Dr /Mr/Mrs/Ms
who will be responsible for the security and confidentiality of my Personal Development Plan, whilst in his/her care.
This permission has been granted on the strict understanding that he/she will not copy any part of my Personal Development Plan, nor divulge any information contained therein, to another party.

Signed: ....
(Submitting GP/PHCT)

Name

Address

Date

Signed: ....
(Assessor)

Date

Appendix 2: Websites

We do not endorse any of the organisations listed in this zone, and we cannot accept any responsibility for any dealings practices may have with any of the organisations listed.

Some organisations change their website periodically, and this can result in links to their website not working properly.

Association for the Study of Medical Education (ASME)	www.asme.org.uk/
Association of British Pharmaceutical Industry	www.abpi.org.uk
Association of Independent Specialist Medical Accountants	http://www.aisma.org.uk/about.asp
Association of Managers in General Practice	www.ihm.org.uk
Association of Medical Secretaries, Practice Managers, Administrators and Receptionists (AMSPAR)	www.amspar.co.uk/frameset.htm
Audit Commission	www.audit-commission.gov.uk
Bandolier	www.jr2.ox.ac.uk/bandolier/
British Medical Association	www.bma.org.uk/
BMJ Appraisal Site Evidence Based Learning Resources	www.bmjlearning.com
BMJ Careers	www.bmjcareers.com/cgi-bin/ section.pl?sn=home
British Association of Medical Managers	www.bamm.co.uk/
British Council (Health)	www.britishcouncil.org/ governance-health-contact-us.htm
British Journal of General Practice	www.rcgp.org.uk/journal/
British Medical Journal	www.bmj.com/
British National Formulary	http://bnf.org/bnf/
British Nursing Association	www.bna.co.uk
Caldicott	www.publications.doh.gov.uk/ipu/ confiden
Cambridge Dictionary On-Line	http://dictionary.cambridge.org/
Central Office for Research Ethics Committee	www.corec.org.uk/
Centre for Evidence Based Medicine	www.cebm.net/

Centre for Innovation in Primary Care (CIPC)	www.innovate.org.uk
Chartered Institute of Personnel and Development	www.cipd.co.uk
Citizens Advice Bureau	www.citizensadvice.org.uk/
Client-Focused Evaluations Program (CFEP)	www.cfep.net/
Clinical Audits – Options	www.nosa.org.uk/information/audit/options.htm
Clinical Governance Bulletin	www.rsmpress.co.uk/cgb.htm
Clinical Governance Support Team	www.cgsupport.nhs.uk/
Clinical Terminology Browser	www.nhsia.nhs.uk/terms/pages
Cochrane Centre	www.cochrane.co.uk
Commission for Patient and Public Involvement in Health (CPPIH)	www.cppih.org/index.html
Commission for Social Care Inspections (CSCI)	www.csci.org.uk/
Commission of Health Improvement (CHI)	www.chi.nhs.uk
Commission of Healthcare Audit and Inspection – CHAI (previous name for Healthcare Commission)	www.healthcarecommission.org.uk
Control of Substance Hazardous to Health (COSHH)	www.hse.gov.uk/coshh/index.htm
Council for the Regulation of Health Care Professionals	www.crhp.org.uk
Critical Appraisal Skills Programme (CASP)	www.phru.nhs.uk/casp/casp.htm
Data Protection Act 1998	www.hmso.gov.uk/acts/acts1998/19980029.htm
Department of Health (DoH)	www.doh.gov.uk
Determining Skill Mix: Practical Guidelines for Managers and Health Professionals	www.moph.go.th/ops/hrdj/hrdj10/special102.htm
Disability Discrimination Act	www.disability.gov.uk/dda/
Doctors Appraisal/Revalidation	www.appraisaluk.info
Doctors Net UK	www.doctors.net.uk/
Doctors Revalidation	www.revalidationuk.info
DoH: Appraisal Website	www.dh.gov.uk/
DoH: Publications and Statistics	www.dh.gov.uk/PublicationsAndStatistics/fs/en
Drugs and Therapeutics Bulletin	www.dtb.org.uk/dtb/
Edgecumbe Consulting – 360degrees	www.edgecumbe.com/edge/
Education for Primary Care	www.radcliffe-oxford.com/epc
Effective Health Care	www.rsmpress.co.uk/ehc.htm
E-learning Centre	www.e-learningcentre.co.uk/eclipse/index.html

Electronic Quality Information for Patients (EQUIP)	www.equip.nhs.uk/
European Computer Driving Licence (ECDL)	http://www.ecdl.com/main/ index.php
European Medicines Evaluation Agency	www.emea.eu.int/
Evidence Based Healthcare and Public Health	www.harcourt-international.com/ journals/ebhc/
Evidence Based Medicine (EBM)	www.cebm.net/
Evidence Based Purchasing	www.jr2.ox.ac.uk/bandolier/ band11/b11-7
Expedition Medicine	www.voyageconcepts.co.uk/ expelist.htm
Exploring New Roles in Practice (ENRiP)	www.shef.ac.uk/snm/research/ enrip/
First Practice Management	www.firstpracticemanagement. co.uk/
Flexible Career Scheme	www.flexiblecareersscheme.nhs.uk
Freedom of Information Act 2000	www.foi-uk.org/about_foi.html
General Medical Council (GMC)	www.gmc-uk.org
General Practice Finance Corporation	www.gpfc.co.uk/
GMS Contract	www.doh.gov.uk/gmscontract/ infotech.htm
Good Practice Guidelines (GPC)	www.doh.gov.uk/gpepr/ guide lines.pdf
GP Appraisal Site	www.gpappraisal.nhs.uk
Health and Safety Commission	www.hse.gov.uk/
Health Care Commission (HCC)	www.healthcarecommission.org.uk www.cgsupport.org
Health Development Agency	www.hda-online.org.uk/
Health Professions Council	www.hpc-uk.org
Health Protection Agency	www.hpa.org.uk
Health Service Journal	www.hsj.co.uk/nav?page=hsj
Health Service Ombudsman	www.ombudsman.org.uk/hse/
Healthy Living Centres	www.nof.org.uk
Honey and Mumford Learning Styles	www.peterhoney.com/product/ brochure
Independent Complaints Advocacy Services (ICAS)	www.dh.gov.uk
Institute of Health Service Managers	www.ihm.org.uk/
Integrated Care Network	www.integratedcarenetwork.gov.uk
International Health Exchange	www.ihe.org.uk
Joint Committee on Postgraduate training for General Practice (JCPTGP)	www.jcptgp.org.uk/
Journal of Evidence Based Medicine	www.ebm.bmjjournals.com/
Journal of Family Practice	www.jfponline.com/default.asp
Kennedy Report	www.bristol-inquiry.org.uk
King's Fund	www.kingsfund.org.uk

Lancet	www.thelancet.com/
Liberating the Talents	www.dh.gov.uk/assetRoot/ 04/07/62/50/04076250.pdf
McMasters University Canada	www.mcmaster.ca/
Medecins Sans Frontieres	www.doctorswithoutborders.org
Medical Defence Union (MDU)	www.the-mdu.com/
Medical Management Services	www.medman.co.uk/pcn/index.htm
Medical Protection Society (MPS)	www.mps.org.uk
Medical Research Council	www.mrc.ac.uk
Medicines and Healthcare Products Regulatory Agency	www.mhra.gov.uk
Medline	www.medlineplus.gov/
Mental Health Act 1983	www.dh.gov.uk/ PublicationsAndStatistics/ Legislation/ActsAndBills/
MeReC Bulletins	www.npc.co.uk/merec_index.htm
Merlin	www.merlin.org.uk
Modernising Medical Careers	www.mmc.nhs.uk
National Association of Clinical Tutors	www.nact.org.uk/
National Association of Patient Participation	http://www.napp.org.uk/
National Association of Primary Care Educators	www.napce.net
National Association of GP Tutors	
National Association of Sessional GPs – NASGP (formerly known as the National Association of Non Principals – NANP)	www.nasgp.org.uk
National Association of GP Co-operatives	www.nagpc.org.uk/
National Clinical Assessment Authority	www.ncaa.nhs.uk
National Counselling Service for Sick Doctors	www.ncssd.org.uk/
National Electronic Library for Health	www.nelh.nhs.uk
National Institute for Clinical Excellence (NICE)	www.nice.org.uk
National Knowledge Service	www.nks.nhs.uk
National Office for GP Recruitment	www.gprecruitment.org.uk/
National Office for Summative Assessment for GP training	www.nosa.org.uk
National Patient Safety Agency	www.npsa.nhs.uk
National Primary and Care Trust Development Programme	www.natpact.nhs.uk
National Primary Care Research and Development Centre	www.npcrdc.man.ac.uk
National Service Framework (NSF)	www.publications.doh.gov.uk/nsf/
National Treatment Agency (Substance Misuse)	www.nta.nhs.uk/

NHS Appraisal Toolkit   www.appraisals.nhs.uk/menu.html

NHS Careers Online   www.nhscareers.nhs.uk/index.html

NHS Centre for Reviews and Dissemination   www.york.ac.uk/inst/crd

NHS Complaint Procedure   www.nhs.uk/england/ aboutTheNHS/ complainCompliment.cmsx

NHS Confederation   www.nhsconfed.org/gmscontract

NHS Direct   www.nhsdirect.nhs.uk

NHS in England – Gateway   www.nhs.uk/england/default.aspx

NHS Individual Learning Accounts   www.dh.gov.uk/ PolicyAndGuidance/ HumanResourcsAndTraining/ LearningAndPersonal Development/

NHS Information Authority   www.nhsia.nhs.uk

NHS Jobs   www.jobs.nhs.uk

NHS Leadership Centre   www.modern.nhs.uk

NHS Litigation Authority   www.nhsla.com

NHS Magazine   www.nhs.uk/nhsmagazine/ default.asp

NHS Modernisation Agency   www.modern.nhs.uk

NHS Patient Survey Programme Advice Centre   www.nhssurveys.org

NHS Pensions Agency   www.nhspa.gov.uk/index.cfm

NHS Plan   www.dh.gov.uk

NHS Professionals   www.nhsprofessionals.nhs.uk

NHS Walk-In Centres   www.nhs.uk/England/ noAppointmentNeeded/ walkinCentres/default.aspx

Nurse Prescribing   www.doh.gov.uk/nurseprescribing

Nursing and Midwifery Council   www.nmc-uk.org

OECD Paper 'Skill mix and Policy Change in the Workforce'   www.oecd.org/dataoecd/30/28/ 33857785.pdf

Open University   www.open.ac.uk

Out of Hours   www.out-of-hours.info/ index. php?pid=10

Patient Advice and Liaison Service (PALS)   www.nelh.nhs.uk/pals/

Patient Association   www.patients-association.com

Patient Concern   www.patientconcern.org.uk

Patient Support Groups   www.patient.co.uk

Pay Review Bodies   www.dh.gov.uk

Pharmaceutical Industry Competitiveness Taskforce   www.advisorybodies.doh.gov.uk/ pictf/

Phased Evaluation Plan (PEP)   www.rcgp-scotland.org.uk/ products/pep

Postgraduate Medical Education and Training Board (PMETB)   www.pmetb.org.uk/pmetb

Prescription Pricing Authority (PPA)   www.ppa.nhs.uk

Primary Care Information Services	www.primis.nhs.uk
Primary Care Research Network	www.ukf-pcrn.org
Quality Assurance Agency for Higher Education	www.qaa.ac.uk
Quality Outcomes Framework	www.doh.gov.uk/gmscontract/ qualityoutcomes.pdf
RCGP International Committee	www.rcgp.org.uk/international/ index.asp
READ Codes	www.equip.ac.uk/readCodes/docs/ index.html
Research and Development Networks in the NHS	www.rdforum.nhs.uk/
Research Journals – Subscriptions	http://juno.ingentaselect.com/vl= 5286832/cl=67/nw=1/rpsv/real page/contents.htm
Royal College of General Practice	www.rcgp.org.uk
Royal College of Nursing	www.rcn.org.uk
Saving Lives: Our Healthier nation	www.ohn.gov.uk
ScHARR	www.shef.ac.uk
Shipman Enquiry	www.the-shipman-inquiry.org.uk www.ihm.org.uk/ content.asp?PageID=469
Significant Event Auditing	www.projects.ex.ac.uk/sigevent/
Skills for Health	www.skillsforhealth.org.uk
Teamwork and Skill Mix	www.nelh.nhs.uk/nsf/ inprimarycare/organisational_ devt/teamwork.htm
The Wisdom Centre – Education and Training for the NHS	www.wisdomnet.co.uk/default.asp
Voluntary Services Overseas (VSO)	www.vso.org.uk/
Wanless Report	www.hm-treasury.gov.uk
Workforce Development Confederations	www.nhscareers.nhs.uk/nhs/ workforce.htm
World Family Doctors (WONCA)	www.globalfamilydoctor.com/
World Health Organisation	www.who.int

References and Further Reading

Achterlonie M, Taylor MB (1998) *Taking Control of Learning. A Small Practices' Association Publication*, Haywood.

Attwood M (2004) *Factors That Influenced GPs to Become GP Educationalists*. MSc Dissertation, University of Portsmouth.

Beck RS, Daughtridge R, Sloan PD (2002) Physician–patient communication in the primary care office: a systematic review. *Journal of the American Board of Family Practice*; **15** (1): 25–38.

Benner P (1984) *From Novice to Expert: Excellence and Power in Clinical Nursing Practice*. Addison-Wesley, Harlow.

Bero LA, Grilli R, Gruimshaw JH, Harvey E, Oxman A, Thomson MA (1998) Closing the gap between research and practice: an overview of systematic reviews of interventions to promote the implementation of research findings. *BMJ*; **317**: 465–8.

British Medical Assocation (2004) *New GMS Contract Explained. Focus on Salaried GPs*. British Medical Assocation, London.

Caplan RP (1994) Stress, anxiety and depression in hospital consultants, general practitioners and senior health service managers. *BMJ*; **306**: 1261–3.

Carr W (1995) *For Education: Towards Critical Educational Inquiry*. The Open University Press, Buckingham.

Cartwright S (2003) *'Contract 2003' – A GPs Guide to Earning the Most*. Butterworth Heinemann, Oxford.

Chambers R (1999) *Survival Skills for GPs*. Radcliffe Medical Press, Oxford.

Chambers R, Davies M (1999) *What Stress in Primary Care!* Royal College of General Practitioners, London.

Chambers R, Schrijver E (2001) Making practice-based professional development plans relegant to service needs and priorities. *Education for General Practice*; **12**: 27–33.

Chambers R, Schwartz A, Boath E (2003) *Beating Stress in the NHS*. Radcliffe Medical Press, Oxford.

Chambers R, Wakley G, Field S, Ellis S (2003) *Appraisal for the Apprehensive: A Guide for Doctors*. Radcliffe Medical Press, Oxford.

Chartered Institute of Personnel and Development (2003) *Continuing Professional Development*. Chartered Institute of Personnel and Development, London.

Chief Medical Officer (1998) *A Review of Continuing Professional Development in General Practice*. Department of Health, Leeds.

CIPC (2000) *What Do Practice Nurses Do? A Study of Roles, Responsibilities and Patterns of Work*. CIPC, Sheffield. Also available at www.innovate.org.uk.

Colby M, Parrott A (1999) *Educational Research and Educational Practice*. Fair Way Publications, Exeter.

Coles C (1994) A review of learner-centred education in primary care. *Education for General Practice*; **5**: 19–25.

Cox T (1993) Stress research and stress management: putting theory to work. HSE Contract Research Report No. 61/1993. Health and Safety Executive, Suffolk.

Curtis AJ (1998) *Opinion Leaders in General Practice*. MSc Dissertation, University of Bath.

Curtis, A, While R, Pitts J, Ramsay R, Attwood M, Wood V (2002) An evaluation of the use of a workbook, *Professional Development*: a guide for general practice, in continuing professional development. *Education for Primary Care*; **15**: 39–49.

Davidoff F (1999) In the teeth of the evidence – the curious case of evidence-based medicine. *Mount Sinai Journal of Medicine*; **66**: 75–83.

Department of Health (1999) *Making a Difference: Strengthening the Nursing, Midwifery and Health Visiting Contribution to Health and Healthcare*. Department of Health, London.

Department of Health (2000) *The NHS Improvement Plan*. Department of Health, Leeds.

Department of Health (2001) *Improving Working Lives Standard*. Department of Health, London.

Department of Health (2002a). *Developing Key Roles for Nurses and Midwives: A Guide for Managers*. Department of Health, London.

Department of Health (2002b) *GP Returners and Flexible Career Scheme for GPs*. Department of Health, Leeds.

Department of Health (2002c) *'Liberating the Talents' Helping Primary Care Trusts and Nurses to Deliver the NHS Plan*. Department of Health, London.

Dixon DM, Sweeney KG, Pereira Gray DJ (1999) The physician healer: ancient magic or modern science? *British Journal of General Practice*; **49**: 309–12.

Epstein RM (1999) Mindful practice. *JAMA*; **282**: 833–9.

Eraut M (1994) *Developing Professional Knowledge and Competence*. Falmer Press, London.

Eve R (2003) *PUNs and DENs. Discovering Learning Needs in General Practice*. Radcliffe Medical Press, Oxford.

Fish D, Coles C (1998) *Developing Professional Judgement in Health Care: Learning through the Critical Appreciation of Practice*. Butterworth Heinemann, Oxford.

Freidson E (1994) *Professionalism Reborn. Theory, Prophecy and Policy*. Policy Press, Bristol.

Gawande A (2002) *Complications: A Surgeon's Notes on an Imperfect Science*. Profile Books, London.

General Medical Council (1993) *Tomorrow's Doctors: Recommendations on Undergraduate Medical Education*. General Medical Council, London.

Golby M, Parrott A (1999) *Educational Research and Educational Practice*. Fairway Publications, Exeter.

Good Medical Practice (2001) *GMC – Protecting Patients, Guiding Doctors*. GMC, London.

Good Practice Guidelines for General Practice Electronic Patient Records (2003). Department of Health & RCGP, London.

Greco M, Francis W, Buckly J, Bronwlea A, McGovern J (1998) Real-patient evaluation of communication skills teaching for GP registrars. *Family Practice*; **15** (1): 51–7.

Hall M, Dwyer D, Lewis T (1999) *The GP Training Handbook* (3rd edn). Blackwell Science, Oxford.

Hastie A (2002) An assessment of the GP Retainer Scheme. *Education for Primary Care*; **13**: 233–8.

Hiss RG, MacDonald R, Davis WK (1978) Identification of physician educational influentials in small community hospitals. *Proceedings Seventh Annual Conference in Research in Medical Education*; **17**: 283–8.

Honey P, Mumford A (2000) *The Manual of Learning Styles.*

House of Commons Health Committee (December 2003) *Building on the Best: Choice, Equity and Responsiveness in the NHS.* House of Commons Health Committee, London.

House of Commons Health Committee (July 2003) *Patient and Public Involvement in the NHS: 7th report of session 2002–3, HC697.* House of Commons Health Committee, London.

Kolb DA (1985) *Experiential Learning.* Prentice Hall, London.

Lave J, Wenger E (1991) *Situated Learning Legitimate Peripheral Participation.* Cambridge University Press, Cambridge.

Lomas J (1993) Teaching old (and not so old) docs new tricks: effective ways to implement research findings. Working paper 93–94. McMaster University Centre for Health Economics and Political Analysis, McMaster University.

Martin D, Harrison P, Joesbury H, Wilson R (2001) *Appraisal for GPs.* University of Sheffield, Sheffield.

Neighbour R (1992) *The Inner Apprentice.* Kluwer Academic Press, London.

NHS (1998a). *A First Class Service: Quality in the new NHS.* Department of Health, London.

NHS (1998b) *GP Retainer Scheme.* Health Service Circular 1998/01. Department of Health, London.

NSH (2001) *NHS Professionals: Flexible Organisations, Flexible Staff.* Health Service Circular 2001/002. Department of Health, London.

Nursing and Midwifery Council (2002) *Code of Professional Conduct.* Nursing and Midwifery Council, London.

O'Connell S (1992) *A Handbook of Non Principals in General Practice.* The Limited Edition Press, Southport.

Pederson TJ (1994) Randomised trial of cholesterol lowering in 4444 patients with coronary heart disease: the Scandinavian Simvastatin Survival Study (4S). *Lancet;* **344**: 1383–9.

Pendleton DA, Schofield TPC, Tate PHL, Havelock PB (2003) *The New Consultation: Developing Doctor – Patient Communication.* The Open University Press.

Picker Institute (2005) *Is the NHS Getting Better or Worse.* Picker Institute, Europe. Also available at http://www.pickereurope.org/Filestore/PressReleases/Press_release_Is_the_NHS_getting_better_or_worse_18_April_05.pdf.

Piercey MI, Waymouth VW (1998) *Managing Performance Distractors Self-Evaluation.* College of Physicians and Surgeons of British Columbia, Vancouver.

Pitts J (1994) Audience involvement in a general practice 'refresher course' – the sharing of 'wants and needs'. *Education for General Practice;* **5**: 190–8.

Pitts J, Curtis A, While R, Holoway I (1999) Practice professional development plans: general practititoners' perspectives on proposed changes in general practice education. *British Journal of General Practice;* **49** (449):959–62.

Pitts J, Vincent S (1995) The higher professional education course in Wessex – the first year. *Education for General Practice;* **6**: 157–62.

Pringle M (1999) The inter-relationship between continuing professional development, clinical governance and revalidation for individual general practitioners. *Journal of Clinical Governance;* **7**: 102–5.

Ramsey PG, Wenrich MD, Carline JD, Invi TS, Larson EB, Loberts JP (1993)Use of peer rating in evaluating physicians performance. *JAMA;* **268**(13):1655–60.

Rosenberg W, Donald A (1995) Evidence-based medicine: an approach to clinical problem solving. *BMJ;* **310**: 1122–6.

Royal College of General Practitioners (1993) Portfolio based learning in general practice. Occasional paper no. 63. Royal College of General Practitioners, London.

Royal College of General Practitioners (1994) Education and training for general practice. Policy Statement 3. Royal College of General Practitioners, London.

Royal College of General Practitioners (1995) Significant event suditing: a study of the feasibility and potential of case-based auditing in primary medical care. Occasional paper no. 70. Royal College of General Practitioners, London.

Royal College of General Practitioners (1999) Clinical governance: practical advice for primary care in England and Wales. Royal College of General Practitioners, London.

Rughani A (2001) GP appraisal and revalidation based on the personal development plan. *Journal of Clinical Governance;* **9**: 175–9.

Sackett DL, Richardson WS, Rosenberg W, Haynes RB (1997) *Evidence Based Medicine: How to Practice and Teach EBM.* Churchill Livingstone, London.

Scally G, Donaldson L (1998) Clinical governance and the drive for quality improvement in the new NHS in England. *BMJ;* **317**: 61–5.

ScHARR (1999) *Developing New Roles in Practice – An Evidence Based Guide.* School of Health and Related Research, University of Sheffield, Sheffield.

Schön D (1984) *The Reflective Practitioner.* Basic Books, New York.

SCOPME (1998a). *Continuing Professional Development for Doctors and Dentists: Recommendations for Hospital Consultant CPD and Draft Principles for All Doctors and Dentists.* Standing Committee on Postgraduate Medical and Dental Education, London.

SCOPME (1998b) *Supporting Doctors and Dentists at Work: An Enquiry into Mentoring.* Standing Committee on Postgraduate Medical and Dental Education, London.

SCOPME (1999) *Doctors and Dentists: The Need for a Process of Review.* Standing Committee on Postgraduate Medical and Dental Education, London.

Secretary of State for Health (1997) *The New NHS, Modern and Dependable.* Department of Health, London.

Stead J, Sweeney G (2001) *Significant Event Audit: A Focus for Clinical Governance.* Kingsham Press, Chichester.

Stewart MA (1995). Effective physician – patient communication and health outcomes: a Review. *Canadian Medical Association Journal;* **152** (9): 1423–33.

Tate P (2002) *The Doctor's Communication Handbook.* Radcliffe Press, Oxford.

The NHS in England (2004/5). *Pocket Guide.* NHS Confederation, England.

The NHS Plan (2000) *A Plan for Investment, A Plan for Reform.* Stationary Office, London.

Thomsen OO, Wulff HR, Martin A, Singer PA (1993) What do gastroenterologists in Europe tell cancer patients? *Lancet;* **341**: 473–6.

Vassilas CA, Donaldson J (1998) Telling the truth: what do general practitioners say to patients with dementia or terminal cancer? *British Journal of General Practice;* **48**: 1081–2.

Walker M, Whincup PH, Shaper AG (2002) Cohort profile: The British Regional Heart Study 1975–2004. *International Journal of Epidemiology;* **33**: 1185–92.

Wensing M, van de Vleuten C, Grol R, Felling A (1997) The reliability of patients' judgement of care in general practice: how many questions and patients are needed? *Quality in Health Care;* **6**: 80–85.

While R, Pitts J, Jones P, Ager P, Rowlands S (1998) Education, audit and active learning: making the links? *Education for General Practice;* **9**: 22–9.

Wilkinson E, Bosanquet A, Salisbury C, Hasler J, Bosanquet N (1999) Barriers and facilitators to the implementation of evidence based medicine in general practice: a qualitative study. *European Journal for General Practice;* **5**: 66–70.

Zurn P, Dal Poz M, Stilwell B, Adams O (2002) Imbalances in the health workforce. Briefing paper. World Health Organization, Geneva.

Index

action plan. *See also* PPDP
   creating, 68–70
activists, 80, 81
additional services, 15–16. *See also* enhanced services;
     essential services; funding streams; practice
   cervical screening, 16
   child health surveillance, 16
   childhood immunisations and boosters, 15
   contraceptive services, 16
   curettage, cautery and cryotherapy, 15
   maternity services (non-intrapartum), 16
   vaccinations and immunisations, 15
administrative audit, 113
   example of, 113
appraisal, 93–106
   GP NHS, 93–97
      GMC, 94
      interview, 95–97
      NHS response line, 94
      preparation, 94
      RCGP, 94
   PHCTs, 97–102
      360 degrees appraisal, 97
      direct line manager appraisal, 97
      documentation, 99
      funding criteria, 99
      GP, 98
      preparation for, 98
      principles of, 97
      process, 98
      purpose of, 97
      training, 98
assessment
   individual skills (clinical), 84–85
   individual skills (non-clinical), 86–87
   team skills, 87–91
audit, 107–130
   administrative, 113
      example of, 113
   CASP, 109–113
   PACT prescribing, 124–127
   performance indicators, 128
      management of, 164
      NSF, 128
      PI as, 129
      QOF, 128
      role of PCO, 128
      vs. competence, 163
   practice, 113–114
      example of, 113–114
   primary care R&D, 107
   R&D in primary care, 107
   referral data, 122
   self-audit, 142
      benefits, 115
      clinical governance, 115
      educational needs, 116
      recording a significant event, 117
      QOF, 115
away days, 74–76. *See also* PHCT
   ground rules, 76
blind spots, 150. *See also* PDP
   clinical skills, 150

   local and national priorities, 150
   new developments in primary care, 150
   personal skills, 150

BMJ, 96
BNF (British National Formulary), 124
brainstorming, 77–78

cardiac arrest, 154–155
career pathways, 180. *See also* PDP
   GP
      retainer and flexible career schemes, 183
      trainer, 185
   GPSI, 182
   job sharing, 182
   portfolio careers, 181
   sabbatical in general practice, 185
   sessional doctors, 180
   teaching PCO, 182
   working in other countries, 186
      expedition medicine, 186
      RCGP international committee, 186
      relief work, 186
caring professionals, 6, 7
CASP. *See* Critical Appraisal Skills Programme
cautery, 15. *See also* additional services
cervical screening, 16
CFEP, 104
child health surveillance, 16. *See also* additional services
chronic obstructive pulmonary disease, 128
Citizens Advice Bureau, 13
clinical effectiveness, 109, 110
clinical governance, 3, 4, 12, 17–20. *See also* PCOs
   clinically effective, 19
   competent staff, 18
   CPD, 4
   evidence sharing, 109
   GP practices, 18
   information systems, 19
   National Institute of Clinical Excellence, 20
   nGMS, 17
   NHS organisations, 4, 17
   patients support and involvement, 18
   PGEA, 4
   quality of care, 17
   risk reduction, 18
   staff support, 18
   transparency in, 128
clinical skills, 105, 150, 153
Clinical Terminology Browser
   TRISET, 23
CMO, 4
   interested parties
      NHS, 4
      patients, 4
      profession, 4
commissioned services, 10. *See also* PCO
communication skills, 151–152
complaints
   dealing, 31
   learning, 31
      MDU, 31
   NHS complaint procedure, 31

PHCT, 31
practice-based, 30–31
consultation, 144. *See also* educational needs
conflicts in
data entry vs. caring, 155
consulting room layout, 156
problem-oriented patient records, 156
SOAP, 156
recording of information, 156, 157
contraceptive services, 16. *See also* additional services
COPD. *See* chronic obstructive pulmonary disease
coping mechanisms, 163
COSHH. *See* Control of Substances Hazardous to Health
CPD (continuing professional development), 4, 43
challenges in probity, 40
clinical governance, 4
Colleague Feedback Evaluation Tool (CFEP), 104
CPD intervetions, 8
GP, 184
NHS, 4
practice nurse, 43
Critical Appraisal Skills Programme, 109. *See also* audit
clinical effectiveness, 109
workshop, 110
cryotherapy, 15. *See also* additional services
curettage, 15
deanery structure, local, 13
NHSMA, 13
secondary care trusts, 13

defibrillation, 154. *See also* PDP
360 degrees feedback, 103–105. *See also* appraisals
benefits of, 103
CFEP, 104
developmental purposes, 105
disadvantages of, 105
for doctors, 103
Edgecumbe Consulting Group, 104
GMC, 103
GP, 103
health service, 103
implementation of, 104
Department of Health, 8, 184. *See also* NHS
appraisal, 94
liberating the talents, 41
SHA, 9
developmental needs, 174–186. *See also* educational needs
DISQ (Doctors' Interpersonal Skills Questionnaire), 29
distractors, 162–164
DoH. *See* Department of Health
DoH appraisal website, 94
dynamising factor, 17. *See also* pension

EBM. *See* evidence-based medicine
Edgecumbe Consulting Group, 104
education and PCOs, 12. *See also* practice
education and practice, 12–13
local deanery structure, 13
NHSMA, 13
secondary care trusts, 13
RCGP, 13
RCN, 13
educational needs, 144–186. *See also* developmental needs
identification of
blind spots, 150
clinical skills, 150
communication skills, 151–152
consultation, 144
conflicts in, 155
consulting room layout, 156
medical ethics, 153
phased evaluation plan, 150
problem-oriented patient records, 156
recording of information, 157

resuscitation, 154–155
sticky moments, 144
stress, 158–164
meeting educational and developmental needs, 174–186
career pathways, 180
HPE, 179
keeping up to date, 178–179
learning goal, 176
learning groups, 178
learning need, 175
learning skills, 174
learning style, 174
mentoring, 177
reflection, 175
working in other countries, 186
enhanced services, 16. *See also* additional services; essential services; funding streams; practice
direct, 16
local, 16
national, 16
ENRiP. *See* exploring new roles in practice
ePFIP. *See* prescribing and financial information for practices electronically
essential services, 15. *See also* additional services; enhanced services; funding streams; practice
evidence-based medicine, 5, 109
management of common disease, 108
exception coding, 22. *See also* nGMS
expedition medicine, 186

feedback, 28–30. *See also* patient
Doctors' Interpersonal Skills Questionnaire, 29
General Practice Assessment Questionnaire, 29
good relationships, 30
Improving Practice Questionnaire, 29
personal development planning, 29–30
postal surveys, 29
practice and team planning, 30
results of, 29
surveys, 28, 29
First Class Service (NHS, 1998), 8
Flexible Career Scheme, 183, 184. *See also* GP Retainer Scheme
funding streams, 15. *See also* nGMS
global sum (GS), 15
minimum practice income guarantee (MPIG), 15
PCO, 15

General Medical Council (GMC), 6, 28, 103
General Practice Assessment Questionnaire, 29
General Practice Questionnaire, 166–172
General Practice Education Committee, 185
global sum, 15
GMC, 28, 103. *See also* appraisal
360 degrees feedback, 103
good medical practice, 104
GP (general practitioner), 37–38, 73, 153
360 degrees feedback, 103
benefits of, 103
CFEP, 104
developmental purposes, 105
disadvantages of, 105
for doctors, 103
GMC, 103
health service, 103
implementation of, 104
accountable to
GMC, 37
NHS, 37
PCOs, 37
appraisal, 93–97
appraisal training, 98
CFEP, 104
complaint dealing, 31
Edgecumbe Consulting Group, 104

health care decisions, 107
leadership, 38–40
PACT, 124
patient feedback, 28
PDP, 137
personal development planning, 29
PHCT, 37, 38
portfolio careers, 181
registrar, 185
retainer, 183
Retainer Scheme, 183
revalidation, 94
surgery, 10
trainer, 185
GP NHS
    appraisal, 93–97
    revalidation, 96
GP practices
    accessible and responsive care, 18
    care environment and amenities, 18
    clinical and cost effectiveness, 18
    governance, 18
    patient focus, 18
    public health, 18
    safety, 18
GP Retainer Scheme, 183, 184. See also Flexible Career
        Scheme
GPAQ. See General Practice Assessment Questionnaire
GPSI (GPs with special interest), 182
    PCO, 182
GS. See global sum

health care
    advancement in, 10
HNA (health needs assessment), 52–72
    action plan, creation, 66
    benefits of, 52
    identifying top health problems, 56
    new priorities, 69
    planning interventions, 62
    practice population key features, 54
    practice population profile, 52
    prioritizing the list, 60
Honey and Mumford, 80
    activists, 80
    pragmatists, 81
    reflectors, 81
    theorists, 81
HPE (higher professional education), 179
    courses, 179
    development, 179
    structure of courses, 179

ICAS. See Independent Complaints Advocacy Services
ILAs (Individual Learning Accounts), 40
immunisations, childhood, 15. See also additional services
Independent Complaints Advocacy Services, 28
information systems, effective use of, 19
interventions planning, 62, 64
IPQ (Improving Practice Questionnaire), 29, 30. See also
        patients, feedback

JCPTGP (Joint Committee on Postgraduate Training for
        General Practice), 183
job sharing, 182

keeping up to date, 178–179

LDP. See local delivery plan
leadership, GP, 38. See also GP
    PCO, 39
learning
    from complaints, 31
    goal, 176

groups, self-directed, 178
highlights, 137, 140, 141
method, 175
need, 175
skills, 174
style, 174
    Honey and Mumford, 80
learning needs
    general, 175
    identification of, 129, 174
    specific, 175
liberating the talents, 41. See also DoH
    clinical role development, 41
    securing better care, 42
    service planning, 41
local delivery plan, 52–72
    PCO, 52

managing performance distractor self-evaluation, 164
maternity services (non-intrapartum), 16. See also
        additional services
MDU (Medical Defence Union), 31, 32
medical ethics, 153. See also educational needs
mentoring, 177. See also PDP
MPIG. See minimum practice income guarantee

National Health Service Modernisation Agency, 8, 13.
        See also NHS and SHAs
National Institute of Clinical Excellence (NICE), 13, 20
National Service Frameworks (NSF), 13, 19–22, 128
    'also-rans', 22
    capacity, 21
    covers
        children, 20
        coronary heart disease, 20
        diabetes, 20
        long-term conditions, 20
        mental health, 20
        National Cancer Plan, 20
        older people, 20
        renal services, 20
    funding, 22
    maximising income, 22
    patient expectation, 20
    prescribing, 21
    secondary care limitations, 21
    staffing expertise, 21
needs
    developmental, 174–186
    educational, 116
    health, 130
    learning, 175
    PCO, 47
nGMS (new GP contract), 3, 15–16, 22, 28
    basic elements of, 15
        additional services, 15–16
        enhanced services, 16
        essential services, 15
        funding streams, 15
    clinical governance, 17
        clinically effective, 19
        competent staff, 18
        CPD, 4
        evidence sharing, 109
        GP practices, 18
        information systems, 19
        National Institute of Clinical Excellence, 20
        NHS organisations, 4, 17
        patient support and involvement, 18
        PGEA, 4
        quality of care, 17
        risk reduction, 18
        staff support, 18
        transparency in, 128

clinical outcomes, 38
 data quality, 22
  READ codes, 23
 exception coding, 22
 patient surveys, 28
 Postgraduate Education Allowance (PGEA), 3
 practice nurses, 40
 quality outcome framework (QOF), 16, 128
  out of hours arrangements, 17
  patient experience, 16
  pensions, 17
  seniority payments, 17
NHS, 8–9
 360 degrees feedback, 103
  benefits of, 103
  CFEP, 104
  developmental purposes, 105
  disadvantages of, 105
  for doctors, 103
  Edgecumbe Consulting Group, 104
  GMC, 103
  GP, 103
  health service, 103
  implementation of, 104
 bean counting 37, 38
 DoH, 8
 funding, 8
 NHSMA, 8
 PALS, 27
 PCO, 52
 pension, 17
 probity, 40
 SHA, 9
 structure of, 9
NHS complaint procedure (2004), 31. *See also*
  patient
 decision, 32
 investigation, 33
 local resolution, 32
 MDU, 32
 panels, 33
 report of investigation, 33
 review procedure, 32
  investigation, 32
  panel hearings, 32
  review, 32
  seniority payments, 17
  out of hours arrangements, 17
NHS organisations, 4, 17. *See also* clinical governance
NHSDirect, 10, 38
NHSMA. *See* National Health Service Modernisation Agency
NICE. *See* National Institute of Clinical Excellence
NMC. *See* Nursing and Midwifery Council
NSFs. *See* National Service Frameworks
Nursing and Midwifery Council, 43

PACT. *See* prescribing analysis and cost
PACT Catalogue
 details of time period, 125
 PCO-employed prescribers, 125
PACT prescribing
 practice formulary and monitor compliance, 124
PACT Standard Report, 124
 national guidance, recent clinical trials data, 124
'painting by numbers' approach, 3
PALS. *See* Patient Advice and Liaison Service
past educational profile, 137. *See also* PDP
patient, 26–34
 advice, 27–28
 concern, 26–27
  GPs, 27
  nGMS, 27
  PALS, 27
  PCO, 27

feedback, 28–30
 Doctors' Interpersonal Skills Questionnaire, 29
 General Practice Assessment Questionnaire, 29
 good relationships, 30
 Improving Practice Questionnaire, 29
 personal development planning, 29–30
 postal surveys, 29
 practice and team planning, 30
 results of, 29
 surveys, 28, 29
Patient Advice and Liaison Service, 27
 and GP practices, 27, 28
 as gateway, 28
 ICAS, 28
 NHS, 27, 28
 NHS complaint procedure (2004), 31–34
 PALS, 27–28
 PCOs, 28
 PCO service information, 28
 practice-based complaints procedure, 30–31
  dealing with complaints, 31
  GP, 31
  learning from complaints, 31
  PHCT, 31
 problem monitoring, 28
patients concern, 26–27
patient expectations, 20
patient feedback, 28–30. *See also* patient
 Doctors' Interpersonal Skills Questionnaire, 29
 General Practice Assessment Questionnaire, 29
 good relationships, 30
 Improving Practice Questionnaire, 29
 personal development planning, 29–30
 postal surveys, 29
 practice and team planning, 30
 results of, 29
 surveys, 28, 29
PCO (primary care organisations)
 and social care, 10
 appraisal training, 98
 as performance indicator, 128
 clinical governance, 12
  clinically effective, 19
  competent staff, 18
  CPD, 4
  evidence sharing, 109
  GP practices, 18
  information systems, 19
  National Institute of Clinical Excellence, 20
  nGMS, 17
  NHS organisations, 4, 17
  patients support and involvement, 18
  PGEA, 4
  quality of care, 17
  risk reduction, 18
  staff support, 18
  transparency in, 128
 collaborative work strategy, 9
 commissioning acute and specialised care, 9
 commissioning decisions, 9
 community health improvement, 9
 consistency in the priorities, 52
 decision-making, 52
 education provision, 12
 health care providers, 10
 LDP, 52
 link with practice, 12
  assessment vs. support dilemma, 12
  clinical governance, 12
  education provision, 12
  medicines management, 12
  nGMS, 12
  performance management vs. development
   dilemma, 12

PMS, 12
 practice-based commissioning, 12
 quality vs. cost dilemma, 12
medical care, 17
medicine management, 12
nGMS, 12
on the spot help, 27
PACT, 124, 125
PALS, 27, 28
population-screening programmes implementation, 9
practice staff, 52
practice-based commissioning, 12
primary and community care services, 9
PRIMIS, 24
READ codes, 24
SHAs, 9
PDP (personal development plan), 3, 4, 12, 29–30, 45,
  47–51, 96, 135–173. *See also* practice
 5-yearly revalidation, 137
 appraisal, 137
 blind spots, 150
  clinical skills, 150
  local and national priorities, 150
  new developments in primary care, 150
  personal skills, 150
 checklists, 142
  challenges, 143
  opportunities, 143
  strengths, 143
  threats, 143
 defibrillation, 154
 different styles of learning, 48
 educational needs identification, 144–173
  sticky moments, 144
 framework for, 137–143
 higher professional education, 179
 learning highlights, 137, 140, 141
 medical ethics, 153
 meeting educational and developmental needs, 174–186
  learning goal, 176
  learning groups, 178
  learning need, 175
  learning skills, 174
  learning style, 174
  mentoring, 177
  reflection, 175
 past educational profile, 137
 phased evaluation plan, 150
 portfolios in learning, 48–49
 reflective practice, 49
 resuscitation, 154–155
 SCOT analysis, 137, 142–143
 self-audit, 137, 142–143
pensions, 17. *See also* Quality and Outcome Framework
PEP. *See* phased evaluation plan
PEP-QB. *See* Phased Evaluation Programme—Question Bank
performance distractor, 164
 management of, 164
 vs. competence, 163
performance indicators, 128–129, 163. *See also* audit
 NSF, 128
 PI as, 129
 QOF, 128
  out of hours arrangements, 17
  patient experience, 16
  pensions, 17
  seniority payments, 17
 role of PCO, 128
personal medical services, 12
PGEA. *See* Postgraduate Education Allowance
phased evaluation plan, 150
 PEP-QB, 151
Phased Evaluation Programme-Question Bank, 151
PHCT. *See* primary health care team

PHCTs appraisals, 97–102. *See also* appraisal
 documentation, 99
 funding criteria, 99
 preparation for, 98
 principles of, 97
 process, 98
 purpose of, 97
 training, 98
  GP, 98
  PCO, 98
 types of
  360 degrees appraisal, 97
  direct line manager appraisal, 97
PIs, 129
PMS. *See* personal medical services
portfolio careers, 181. *See also* GP
PPA. *See* Prescription Pricing Authority
PPDP. *See* practice professional development plan
practice, 12–25. *See also* education and practice
 audit, 113–114
 commissioning, 13
 complaints procedure, 30–31
 enhancement, 24
 link with, 12–14
  Citizens Advice Bureau, 13
  education, 12–13
  local and national organisations, 13
  NHS, 13
  PACT, 13
  PCOs, 12–13
  Prescription Pricing Authority, 13
 national initiatives, 15
  clinical governance, 17–20
  nGMS, 15
  NSFs, 20–22
  QOF, 16
 nurse, 40–43
 population, 58
 PPDP, 52
 professional development plan, 3, 4, 47–72, 131–134
practice audit, 113–114. *See also* audit
 example of, 113–114
practice nurse, 40–43. *See also* primary health care team
 chronic diseases care, 41
 developments, 41
 extended formulary, 42
 prescribing, 42
 professional development for, 43
  CPD, 43
practice population, 58
 action plan, 68
 drug and alcohol abuse, 58
 high elderly population, 58
 HNA, 52
 key features, 56
 new priorities, 71
 planning interventions, 64
 prioritising the list, 62
 profile of, 54
 top health problems identification, 58
practice professional development plan, 3, 4, 47–72,
  131–134. *See also* personal development plan
 action plan, 66, 68–70
 components of, 131–134
  GP appraisal, 132
  health needs assessment, 132
  local delivery plan, 132
  practice SCOT analysis, 132
 creating an action plan, 68
 creating profile of practice population, 54
  identification of top health problems in your
   practice, 58
 education and development, 47
 health needs assessment, 52–72

key features of your practice population, 56
local delivery plans, 52–72
PACT, 125
PCO, 131
PCO needs, 47
PHCT, 131
prioritising action list, 62
planning interventions, 64
practice-based commissioning, 13
practice-based complaints procedure, 30–31
GP, 31
learning from complaints
MDU, 31
PALS, 30
PHCT, 31
pragmatists, 81–82
professional development plan, practice. See practice professional development plan
prescribing, 21
PACT
practice formulary and monitor compliance, 124
prescribing analysis and cost, 13, 124–127
data
PACT Catalogue, 124
PACT Standard Report, 124
expensive prescription medicines, 124
PCO, 124, 125
PPA, 124
PPDP, 125
Prescription Pricing Authority, 13, 124
ePFIP, 125
primary care
ambulance trusts, 10
care trusts, 10
GP, 10
practice and PCOs interface, 10
surgery, 10
mental healthcare trusts, 10
NHS trusts, 10
R&D, 107
Primary Care Information Service, 24
primary care organisations, 3, 12–13
primary health care team, 3, 4, 12, 37–44, 73, 152
appraisal, 97–102
away day, 73–76
ground rules, 76
brainstorming, 77–78
complaints dealing, 31
development, 73–82
GP, 37–38
groups, small, 76, 77
Honey and Mumford, 80
activists, 80
pragmatists, 81
reflectors, 81
theorists, 81
learning profiles, 80
PDPs, 12
PPDP, 12, 131
practice nurses, 40–43, 73
SCOT analysis, 79
secondary care limitations, 21
size of, 74
skill mix, 83–92
PRIMIS
PCO, 24
Primary Care Information Service, 24
probity, 40
professional development, 5–8
clinical governance, 4
enhanced professional self-regulation, 4
life-long learning, 4
professional knowledge, 6–7
Carr's view, 6–7

professional practice, 5–6
natural change in, 7

QMAS. See Quality Management and Analysis System
QOF (Quality and Outcome Framework), 16–17, 23, 37, 128. See also nGMS; practice
out of hours arrangements, 17
patient experience, 16
pensions, 17
dynamising factor, 17
seniority payments, 17

RCGP. See Royal College of General Practitioners
RCGP international committee, 186
RCN. See Royal College of Nurses
READ code. See also nGMS
NHS, 23
PCO, 24
QMAS, 23
TRISET, 23
referral data, 122. See also audit
reflective practice, 49. See also PDP
reflectors, 81
research and audit, 107
resuscitation, 154–155. See also educational needs
retained doctors, 183
revalidation, 3
revalidation, GP NHS, 96
Royal College of General Practitioners, 13, 94, 150.
Royal College of Nurses, 13

ScHARR (School of Health and Related Research), 93
SCOT analysis, 79, 142–143. See also PHCT
screening, cervical, 16
SEA. See significant-event auditing
secondary care limitations, 21
PHCT, 21
self-audit, 142. See also audit
SCOT analysis, 137
services
additional, 15–16
commissioned, 10
contraceptive, 16
enhanced, 16
essential, 15
maternity (non-intrapartum), 16
sessional doctors, 180, 181
SHAs. See Strategic Health Authorities
significant event, 115–121
SEA, 115
significant-event auditing, 114–121.
benefits, 115
clinical governance, 115
educational needs, 116
QOF, 115
recording, 117
skill mix, 83–92. See also primary health care team
advanced beginner, 83
competent, 83
expert, 83
novice, 83
proficient, 83
SOAP, 156
sticky moments, 144–150
Strategic Health Authorities, 8
coherent strategic NHS framework, 8
as DoH and NHS front line link, 9
high-quality performance ensurance, 9
implementation and delivery of NHS plan, 8
national priorities integration, 9
NHS management, 9
and NHSMA, 8
PCOs, 9
performance-manage PCOs, 8

staffing expertise, 21
strategy development, 9
stress, 158–164
    control of, 161
    effects of, 159
    sources of, 159
    symptoms of, 158
        behavioural symptoms, 158
        personal symptoms, 158

substance misuse, 19. *See also* GP
surveillance, child health, 16. *See also* additional services

teaching PCOs, 182
theorists, 81
TRISET, 23

vaccinations, 15. *See also* additional services
5-yearly revalidation, 137. *See also* PDP